Jenny Jones.

# Information Technology for the Caring Professions

# Information Technology for the Caring Professions

## A User's Handbook

*Sydney S. Chellen*
MEd(Kent), BA(Ed), RNT, RCNT, PGCE(FE), RMN, RGN
Senior Lecturer Nursing Studies
Canterbury Christ Church College
Canterbury

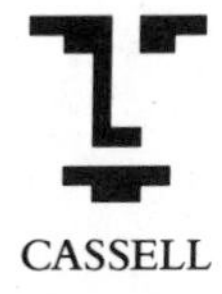

CASSELL

Cassell
Villiers House
41/47 Strand
London WC2N 5JE

387 Park Avenue South
New York
NY 10016-8810



**British Library Cataloguing-in-Publication Data**
A catalogue record for this book is available
from the British Library.

**Library of Congress Cataloging-in-Publication Data**
Chellen, Sydney S.
Information technology for the caring professions: a user's handbook / Sydney S. Chellen.
p. cm.
Includes bibliographical references and index.
ISBN 0-304-33162-7 (hb) : $70.00
ISBN 0-304-33164-3 (pb) : $26.00
1. Medical informatics. 2. Computers. 3. Electronic data processing. I. Title.
[DNLM: 1. Computer Systems—programmed instruction. W26.5 C5161 1995]
R858.C46 1995
610'.285—dc20
DNLM/DLC
for Library of Congress 94-18463
CIP

ISBN 0-304-33162-7 (hb)
0-304-33164-3 (pb)

Designed and typeset by John Hawkins Book Design
Printed and bound in Great Britain by The Bath Press

## Disclaimer

Because the author has no control over the circumstances of use of this handbook and associated workbooks, he cannot assume liability or responsibility for any consequential loss or damage, however caused, arising as a result of carrying out the exercises in the book and associated workbooks. These materials are offered to the purchaser on the basis of this understanding.

All the information in the handbook and related workbooks is believed to be correct at the time of printing. Whenever possible the author will try to assist with any queries.

To my late parents, Georgina, Patricia,
David and Maurice

# Contents

## Acknowledgements

In writing this book I have drawn upon my experience of many years using and exploiting computers as a tool in handling information. However, I am equally indebted to all my colleagues who read the manuscript before publication and generously offered helpful suggestions.

I also wish to express appreciation to all the nursing students who carried out some of the exercises in the book and willingly offered their comments, particularly Mrs Diane Cane.

A special thank you goes to Pat Gordon Smith, Commissioning Editor at Cassell, for her suggestions, words of encouragement and interest in the book.

Finally, I must thank my family, particularly my wife Georgina, for tolerating my sometimes 'intolerable' behaviour and the clacking of my computer keyboard in the early hours of the morning. To them, and all those who have kept my interest in this project, this book is partly due.

# To the reader

## Introduction

Computers are rapidly becoming an integral part of the health care system. These computers are being used by health professionals for a variety of purposes. A short list includes:

- **generating** letters, memos, reports etc.;
- **gathering** and storage of demographic, clinical, and administrative data;
- **recording** of contacts with clients, particularly by community workers, GPs, counsellors;
- **management** of finance and billing;
- **monitoring** of patient vital signs, fluid balance, cardiac arrythmias and so on;
- **calculation** of laboratory results;
- **analysis** of statistical data on admission and discharge, size of case load;
- **scheduling** of appointments;
- **planning** of care.

It will not be long before computers are widely used to generate nursing and medical diagnoses so that health professionals can develop action plans based on these diagnoses.

As the use of computers is growing quickly across the welfare services, all health professionals need to become confident in their use of information technology. A computer should be a tool to help you work more effectively. With the wealth of nursing and health care data now available, it will be an essential learning resource throughout your career. No amount of knowledge or skill is too much. Indeed, when it comes to computers, a little knowledge can waste you a lot of time and in some cases can also be costly.

Like any machine, computers require that you take some time and effort learning to operate them correctly. If, at the moment, you are confused by them or feel you do not know enough, you are not alone. With a little work you will be developing skills that you never thought possible. After working through this book you should be well on your way to peaceful co-existence with computers.

## What is this book about and who should use it?

This handbook on computer technology and its application in health care settings assumes no prior knowledge or skill. It is designed to give you a progressive and thorough understanding of the computer and all its uses. As such, it will also be invaluable to those who have picked up some computer skills on an ad hoc basis. Later units on computer languages and nursing research will be of use to quite advanced computer users. It is written specifically to meet the needs of:

- All students of nursing: Project 2000 nurses, trainee midwives, RNs converting to diploma, Bachelor and Master of Nursing students, those following a path to the Higher Award in nursing.
- Medical students, trainee occupational therapists, trainee physiotherapists, trainee pharmacy technicians.
- Professionals working in the health and welfare

services – be they in hospital or community environments.

## Structure of the book

To make learning and revision as easy as possible, the book has been divided into eleven distinct yet related learning units. It includes the following features:

- self-assessment questionnaires;
- suggested assignments;
- endnotes;
- appendices;
- revision tests;
- glossaries of terms;
- reading list;
- index.

A special feature of the book is that there are two types of boxes appearing on almost every page:

- **Facts boxes** which contain additional useful information.
- **Glossary of terms**. Although basic terms are explained in the text, they also appear alongside in boxes. A complete list of terms is included at the end of the handbook.

Each unit starts with a self-assessment questionnaire so that you can assess your knowledge base. Depending on the percentage score you achieve you will be guided on how best to proceed with this book.

At the end of each unit there are suggested assignments - some are in the form of practical exercises for which you will need a computer with a hard disk and others are in the form of projects, topics for discussions or simply areas for reflection. Each unit ends with a set of learning outcomes. At the end of the book you will find a revision test on all aspects covered in the units together with a comprehensive list of books and articles that you can read to further your understanding and awareness in health care computing.

**Unit 1** gives an overview of computer systems. This unit is purposely short and to the point. It defines a computer and explains some important terms. A short overview of the hardware which makes up a computer system is given. The purpose of the operating system is explained. An assignment to increase your awareness of the types of computer systems and application software available in health care settings is included.

**Unit 2** takes a look at some of the devices that may be connected to a computer and their possible applications in health care settings. The necessary precautions that should be taken with storage devices are itemized and explained. Various exercises appear at the end of this unit. These are offered to help you gain practical experience, so that you can appraise the usefulness of various input and output devices for personal and professional use, and acquire both knowledge and skills.

**Unit 3** details in plain language the various tasks that a computer can do and illustrates how computers and the use of computer networks can be a significant boon to health professionals in the clinical environment (hospital and community centres) and at home.

In **Unit 4** the basic parts of the computer are identified and described. A brief explanation is given of how the computer works, and exercises are included at the end of the unit.

**Unit 5** takes a closer look at computer systems. This is to increase your awareness of the great advances being made in computer technology. The differences between various systems, including laptops, are highlighted. Exercises in this unit are designed to assist the reader to identify personal strengths and weaknesses with regard to computers.

In **Unit 6** some problems and issues associated with computers (such as confidentiality and security of information) are identified and where possible solutions are given. Other related issues associated with computers, such as confidentiality of information stored in computers, security of personal data, rights of data subjects and software copyright are highlighted and where possible solutions are given. Relevant requirements of the Data Protection Act, such as the obligations of data users and the rights of data subjects, are explained. Health problems associated with VDUs are identified and appropriate actions that can be taken in order to minimize the risk of ill-health are suggested. A section about copyright law governing computer programs is also included. The aim of the assignments at the end of this unit is to provide the reader with an opportunity to consider the likely problems with regard to automation of data in hospital settings and the responsibility of health professionals with regard to personal data belonging to patients/clients.

In **Unit 7** an explanation is given of how the Disk Operating System (DOS) manages all the information that is put into the computer. The concept of directories and paths is described. Explanations of how to issue commands to DOS are given, and several exercises are included.

**Unit 8** gives up-to-date information on the continuing development of electronic techniques to make computers more user friendly. The WIMP technique is described. Using 'screen shots', specific areas are explained. The advantages of Windows over DOS are highlighted. A variety of simple practical exercises for using Windows are included.

**Unit 9** explains how to communicate with computers to reduce the frustration of the user when working with these machines. Common errors are highlighted and how they can be avoided is described. A brief description of various computer languages and how they differ is included.

In **Unit 10** research activities are identified. This is followed by an explanation of how the computer can help health professionals with these research activities. Databases relating to research in health care are identified and their contents are briefly described. Statistical packages for analysing nursing data are identified. How a tool for collecting data could be constructed is explained. How data should be prepared for input into the computer for analysis is also explained. Several exercises designed to help the reader use a statistical package for analysis of data are included.

Finally, in **Unit 11** some limitations of computers are identified and how they can be managed is discussed.

## How to use this book

As the book assumes no previous knowledge and builds on knowledge acquired in the previous units, you will get far more out of it if you read each unit in sequence. If you already know something about computers, then you should at least survey each unit before moving on to the next one. The book provides **self-assessment tests**, **learning outcomes** and **assignments** for each unit as well as a **revision test** and a comprehensive **list of books and articles for further reading** at the end. I suggest that you adopt the following steps, which should help you to get the most out of this book.

First answer the questions at the beginning of Unit 1. Decide how confident you feel about the answers you gave and score yourself as suggested. Add up your scores. Then, using the self-rating score-ometer, proceed as follows:

| | |
|---|---|
| 90 to 100 per cent | You could skip this unit, if you are absolutely confident with your answers. |

| | |
|---|---|
| 50 to 89 per cent | You should at least survey this unit. |
| 25 to 49 per cent | You would be well advised to read relevant subsections of this unit. |
| Below 25 per cent | You would benefit from reading the whole unit. |

As you read, make notes as appropriate.

When you reach the end of the unit, look at the suggested assignments. Decide how feasible it is for you to do them, but do make the effort. Remember: no pain, no gain.

Now look at the **Endnote** of that unit. It lists the expected learning outcomes. Ask yourself whether you have achieved them. If not, read through the unit again before moving on to the next.

When you have completed all the units, start answering the questions in the **revision test**. You can check your answers by referring back to the text. Then compare your original scores on the self-assessment tests at the beginning of each unit as they will provide you with a good baseline to see how much you have learnt.

Finally, remember that a book of this size cannot be completely comprehensive. If after you have completed the book, you find yourself talking intelligently about computers, with sufficient interest to do further reading as recommended, then this book will have more than fulfilled its main purpose.

# Self-Assessment Test for Unit 1

## Instructions

Answer the following questions. Decide how confident you feel about each of your answers and mark your score in the column provided or on a piece of paper. The weighting for each question is shown in the right-hand column. When you have answered all the questions, add up your marks. Then look at the scoreometer to determine your rating.

| No. | Question | Expected Score | Actual Score |
|---|---|---|---|
| 1 | What is a computer? | 1 | |
| 2 | What is meant by the following terms: | | |
| | hardware | 1 | |
| | software | 1 | |
| | MS-DOS | 1 | |
| | Application programs | 1 | |
| | CPU | 1 | |
| 3 | What is meant by a computer system? List three types. *(1 mark each)* | 4 | |
| 4 | List the three pieces of hardware that make up a computer system. *(1 mark each)* | 3 | |
| 5 | List three types of operating system. *(1 mark each)* | 3 | |
| 6 | What does the abbreviation VDU stand for? | 1 | |
| 7 | Give two other names for the VDU. *(1 mark each)* | 2 | |
| 8 | What types of computers are in use in health care settings? | 4 | |
| 9 | What software packages are health professionals using to manage health care? | 5 | |
| | **Total score** | **28** | |

## Scoreometer

**26 to 28** You can skip this unit if you are absolutely confident with your answers.
**14 to 25** You should at least survey this unit.
**7 to 13** You would be well advised to read relevant sub-sections of this unit.
**0 to 6** You would benefit from reading the whole unit.

# UNIT 1
# The computer system 1 – an overview

## 1.1 What is a computer?

Consider the following terms for a moment: microcomputer or micro; personal computer or PC; desktop computer or desktop for short. They all mean a piece of equipment that can be operated by a single person and that usually stands on top of a desk. Basically, a computer is a programmable machine that accepts, processes and displays information, while a computer system is a group of interacting parts which operate together to achieve a common end. Different types of computer systems are in existence: mainframes, minicomputers and microcomputers (PCs). (For more information see Unit 5.)

## 1.2 Overview of the computer system

There are two basic aspects of a computer system: the **hardware** and the **software**. The hardware is literally the hard parts that you can touch and consists of the keyboard, monitor and the system unit. The system unit holds the **CPU (central processing unit)**, memory, disk drive(s), ports and video card (Figure 1.1). The software, broadly speaking, refers to the **programs** that provide the driving force of all computing systems.

### GLOSSARY OF TERMS 1

A **computer** is a programmable machine that accepts, processes and displays information/data.

A **computer system** is a group of interacting parts that operate together to achieve a common end.

**Hardware** is the physical or tangible apparatus of a computer system, i.e. all input and output devices.

A **program** is a series of detailed instructions written in a computer language that tells the computer what to do, e.g. a program might tell the computer to sort a list of names alphabetically.

**Software**, broadly speaking, refers to the programs which provide the driving force of all computing systems. There are two types: (a) operating systems software and (b) applications software.

The **CPU** – central processing unit – is the part of a computer that interprets and executes instructions. It is composed of an arithmetic logic chip, a control unit and a small amount of memory.

A **monitor** is a television-like output device for displaying data. Also referred to as a VDU (visual display unit).

**Hardware: the CPU, monitor and keyboard**

The CPU is the heart and soul of a computer and is the place where all the instructions are stored and carried out.

When you communicate with the computer, the **monitor** displays instructions on the screen. The computer uses the monitor screen to send messages and results back to you after interpreting your instructions. The screen may display information in one colour or in several colours. For a colour monitor to display colour, it needs an appropriate video card, which fits inside the system unit. Some video cards enable the monitor to display graphics.

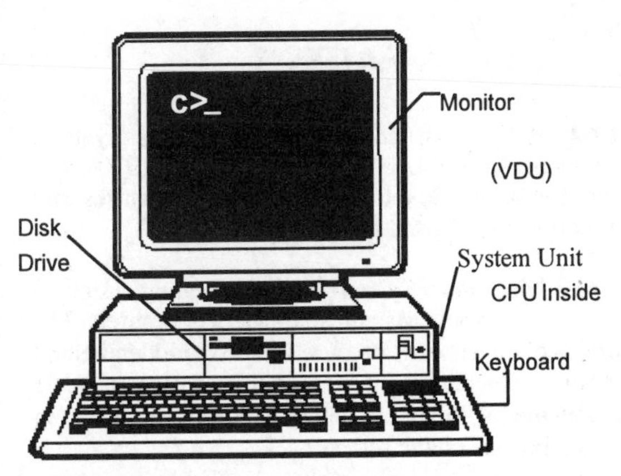


Figure 1.1 A computer system

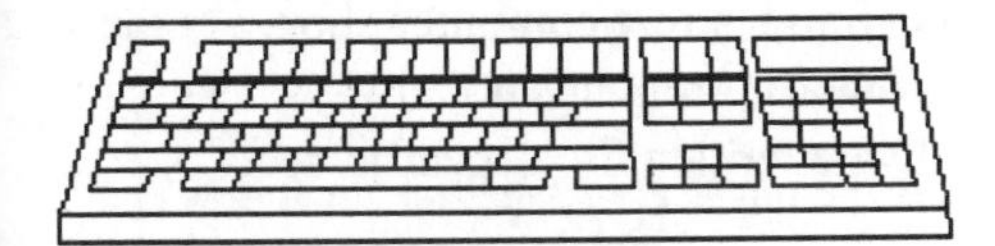

Figure 1.2 The extended keyboard

The **keyboard** is one means by which you communicate with the computer. All keyboards have letter keys, punctuation keys and a spacebar, which resemble the keys on a typewriter. These are used in the same way as on a typewriter. Most keyboards also have numeric and arrow keys, as well as ESC, CTRL, ALT, DEL, ENTER or RETURN and function keys. Examples of function keys are F1, F2, F3 etc.Their location on the keyboard varies according to the type of keyboard, i.e. standard or extended (Figure 1.2). The software determines how they are used.

**Ports**, i.e. sockets, are located at the back of the system unit. They are used for making connections between the computer and other hardware such as the monitor, keyboard, mouse and printer.

**Software: operating system and application programs**

The programs which store the computer's instructions are known as software and there are two main types:

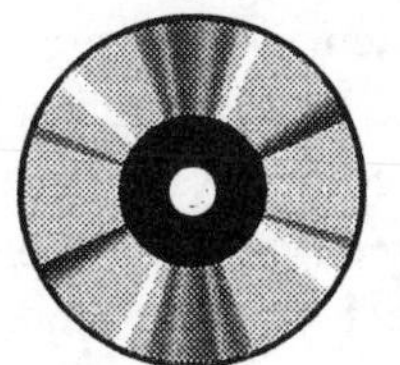

Fig 1.3
A CD-ROM

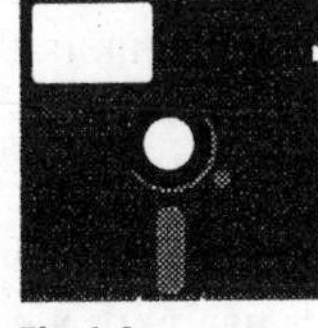

Fig 1.4a
5.25" Floppy disk

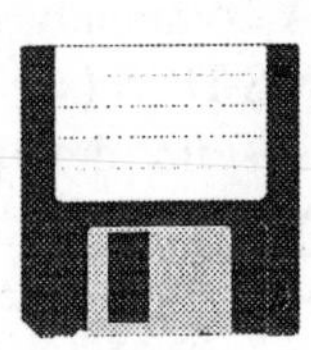

Fig 1.4b
3.5" Floppy disk

- operating system;
- application programs.

The operating system is a piece of software which may be likened to the brain of Frankenstein's monster. Without the operating system – or 'brain' – the computer is nothing but a monster incapable of carrying out any task whatsoever.
However, when you load up the operating system you give the computer an environment which it understands and in which it can function. It is the job of the operating system to follow the user's instructions, such as copying files to **disks** (Figures 1.3 and 1.4), as well as a variety of other 'housekeeping' tasks.

## GLOSSARY OF TERMS 2

An **operating system** is a complex computer program used to control, assist or supervise all other programs that run on a computer system.

**Application programs** are pre-written programs which contain specific instructions to enable the computer to carry out tasks such as word processing or accounting.

A **disk** is a round magnetized plate, usually made of plastic or metal, organized into concentric tracks and pie-slice shaped sectors for storing data. There are a number of different types of disk. See Section 2.5 for more information.

**MS-DOS** is an abbreviation for Microsoft Disk Operating System. Several alternative operating systems are available.

**Ports** are connection points between computers and external devices such as printers.

A commonly used operating system is known as MS-DOS (*see* Unit 7). This is the Disk Operating System developed by a US company called Microsoft and is generally regarded as the worldwide standard. A document prepared and stored on a disk for use with a computer using one type of operating system cannot normally be used by a machine using another operating system (*see* Facts 1).

The **application programs** cannot be run without first loading the operating system. Application programs are pre-written software programs which contain specific instructions to enable the computer to carry out tasks such as word processing or accounting, and are discussed at greater length later on. These programs can be bought ready-written from the local high street computer shop. As there are plenty to choose from it is not always necessary to have software written for a specific need.

### FACTS 1

**UNIX™** is another popular operating system, developed at Bell Laboratories in the early 1970s. The VAX system – found in universities, industries and government departments – uses UNIX.

**Apple Macintosh System 7.** This operating system is used on the Apple Macintosh range of computers. The user will never see it because it is well hidden behind a full graphical user interface which replaces obscure commands with simple manipulations carried out on visual objects on the screen.

## Suggested Assignments

AIMS — To increase your awareness of the types of computer systems and application software available in the clinical environment.*
To orientate you with computer keyboards.

ACTIVITY 1 — During your next working day(s) in your clinical environment, find out and make a list of:
(a) the type(s) of computers in use;
(b) the devices that are connected to the computers;
(c) the software packages that are being used.

ACTIVITY 2 — If you have never used a computer before, find a computer keyboard, and locate on it the following keys: †

(a) the ESCape key;
(b) the ALT key;
(c) the CTRL key;
(d) the RETURN or ENTER key;
(e) the FUNCTION or F keys;
(f) the NUMERIC keys;
(g) the position of the ALPHA keys;
(h) the Cursor control keys.

* This could apply to any unit in which health care activities take place, e.g. hospitals, clinics, health centres, doctors' surgery.
† See Appendix 1 for an explanation of their functions.

## Endnote

Now that you have completed this unit you should be able to:

- define a computer;
- explain the terms hardware, software, CPU, operating system, application programs;
- identify the hardware which forms a computer system;
- name three types of operating system;
- identify and describe the application programs in use in health care;
- recognize different types of computers which can be found in health centres;
- list the common devices that are connected to computer systems in health care.

# Self-Assessment Test for Unit 2

## Instructions

Answer the following questions. Decide how confident you feel about each of your answers and mark your score in the column provided or on a piece of paper. The weighting for each question is shown in the right-hand column. When you have answered all the questions, add up your marks. Then look at the scoreometer to determine your rating.

| No. | Question | Expected Score | Actual Score |
|---|---|---|---|
| 1 | List fourteen precautions that should be taken when handling a floppy disk. *(1 mark each)* | 14 | |
| 2 | List four devices that can be connected to a computer. *(1 mark each)* | 4 | |
| 3 | List eight features that ought to be taken into account when selecting a printer. *(1 mark each)* | 8 | |
| 4 | How does a fax-modem differ from a fax machine? | 2 | |
| 5 | (a) Differentiate between a floppy disk and a hard disk. *(1 mark)*<br>(b) State why it is necessary to format a new disk. *(1 mark)* | 2 | |
| 6 | (a) What are the names of the following devices? *(1 mark each)*<br>(b) What are they used for? | 4 | |
| 7 | (a) What size of disk is this?<br>(b) Identify the following:<br>(i) index hole;<br>(ii) hub;<br>(iii) window;<br>(iv) write protect notch;<br>(v) label. | 6 | |
| | **Total score** | **40** | |

## Scoreometer

**36 to 40** You can skip this unit if you are absolutely confident with your answers.
**20 to 35** You should at least survey this unit.
**10 to 19** You would be well advised to read relevant sub-sections of this unit.
**0 to 9** You would benefit from reading the whole unit.

# UNIT 2
# Computer peripherals and accessories

In addition to the basic computer system, there are computer peripherals, i.e. devices which may be connected to the computer. These include items such as a printer, mouse, modem, scanner and floppy disks.

## GLOSSARY OF TERMS 3

**Peripherals** are various attachments to the computer, e.g. keyboard, monitor, disk drive, printer, mouse.

**Accessories** are materials required for use with the computer.

A **document** is a piece of work with a specific name, performed on a computer for storage and which can be retrieved immediately or at a later date.

## 2.1 Printers

**Daisywheel**

The printing characters of a daisywheel printer are at the tip of thin flexible strips, one to two inches long, and set in a circle.

Printing is restricted to the characters embossed on the daisy wheel, but the wheel can be changed. The wheel rotates until the correct character is positioned in front of a hammer, which strikes the tip of the stalk on which the character is embossed against a ribbon to produce an image of the character.

A daisywheel printer produces print quality similar to that of a typewriter, which makes it suitable for word processing. The printing speed can range from 10 to 80 characters per second (c.p.s.), depending on the make and quality of the printer. Although the print quality is superior to that of a dot matrix printer, the daisywheel printer does not have the ability to produce graphics. Laser printers can produce graphics of excellent quality. They are versatile and, owing to recent price decreases, are becoming a very popular choice for those who require good quality printing.

**Dot matrix**

This is a fairly basic, but quite flexible printer. It can produce text or graphics in the form of a matrix of small dots, with each character formed by a series of pins striking a ribbon. The cheaper printers normally use nine pins to produce one character while the better dot matrix printers use 24 pins to output a much higher quality text, generally almost as good as that produced by a typewriter. This is called NLQ (near letter quality). Dot matrix printers are extremely versatile and are generally used for jobs where the quality of print is not crucial, such as working on particular **documents** during the draft stages. Different print modes, such as condensed, enlarged, underlined and bold, can be selected. The dot matrix printer has a printing speed in the region of 120–150 c.p.s. for NLQ and 250–400 c.p.s. for draft. Some models have multi-colour ribbons for colour printing.

**Laser printers**

These are fast, flexible and sophisticated. A laser printer works on similar principles to a photocopier, using a photosensitive drum, and can produce between four and 20 pages per minute. The quality of the daisywheel is combined with the flexibility of a dot matrix. Laser printers provide very high quality reproduction, including graphics. Using appropriate software, such as a desktop publishing package, business documents, invoices, statements and so on can be printed complete with headings – removing the need for pre-printed stationery.

Laser printers are quickly becoming inexpensive and affordable. Early models cost in the region of £20,000 – 100,000, but they are now available for around £500. A laser printer is an absolute must for graphics or desktop publishing and gives a very high quality look to any computer document.

**Thermal printers**
This type of printer is both quiet in operation and inexpensive. It uses thermal electrosensitive paper which has a thin coating of aluminium over a black- or blue-inked surface. An electric current is passed through a needle on to the paper to produce a spark, which removes a small area of aluminium and exposes the black or blue undersurface.

**Ink jet printers**
Like thermal printers, ink jet printers can be described as the 'poor man's' laser printers. The ink jet printing system prints characters and graphics by firing ink drops at the paper from thin nozzles. The ink is heated in these nozzles, by the application of electrical pulses to the heating elements, producing bubbles that quickly expand and eject the ink. An important feature of this printing system is the simple construction of individual nozzles, which makes the printing mechanism more durable. These printers use a replaceable ink cartridge that contains both the print head and the ink. They are extremely quiet.

The Hewlett-Packard DeskJet550C, for example, is a very close imitation of a laser printer, offering professional quality black and white or colour printing. It can even print on transparencies, although a special type of transparency paper is required with ink jets, and this is not cheap.

## FACTS 2

Printers are available with a wide range of features. The following are some factors than should be considered when selecting a printer:

- compatibility;
- speed;
- column width, i.e. 80 or 136 characters per line;
- colour or black and white printing;
- parallel or serial interface;
- graphics capabilities;
- uni- or bi-directional;
- plain or thermal paper;
- cut sheets or continuous stationery;
- single or varying character pitches;
- price;
- running costs.

Compatibility problems between computers and printers are almost a thing of the past. All the main computer types (Atari ST, Amiga, Archimedes, Apple Macintosh and PC-compatible) have the same printer interfaces: one type is called serial or RS232, while the other is called parallel or Centronics. Printers which have parallel interfaces are better, because data transfer is faster than with those with serial ports.

**Line printers**
Line printers are impact printers. They print a complete line of characters on each revolution. Typical speeds are 200–3000 lines per minute. Line printers are used for high volume printing requirements in mainframe and minicomputer installations (*see* Unit 5). The barrel-type printer has characters embossed around a print barrel while the chain-type has characters embossed on a chain. The barrel or the chain rotates and a hammer prints the required characters.

## 2.2 Mouse

The mouse is a plastic device about the size of a pack of cards and is usually attached to the computer by a long wire which looks like a tail: hence the name. This input device allows you to control the computer without learning how to use the keyboard. On top of the mouse there are one or more buttons which you can press, and usually at the bottom there is a ball that rolls when the mouse is moved on the desk. This action causes a pointer (often drawn as an arrow) to move in a corresponding direction on the computer screen. By pointing the arrow to objects or wording on the screen and clicking one of the buttons on the mouse you can tell the computer to carry out certain activities. Most mice work by rolling the mouse ball across a flat surface (the top of the desk or a cushioned 'mouse pad'). There are different types of mouse, such as trackball mouse, thumb mouse and one-, two- or three-button mouse. Most mice have two buttons. For some application programs, knowing how to use a mouse is a must.

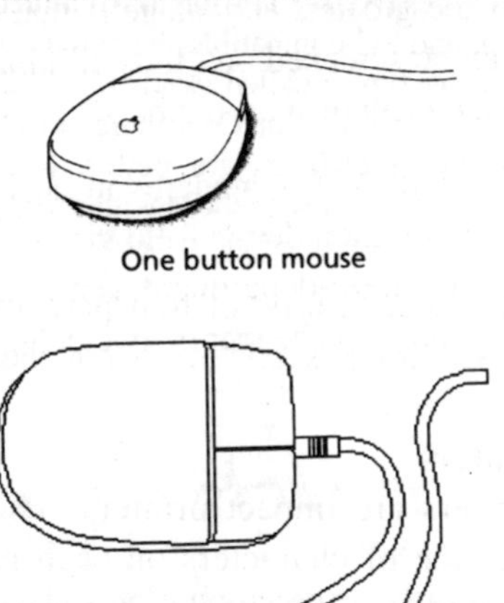

One button mouse

Two button mouse

**Figure 2.1** Two types of mouse

## 2.3 Modem and fax-modem

A modem is a device that enables data to be transmitted between computers over long distances, using either the public telephone network or privately installed fibre-optic cables or radio frequencies. It enables one computer to talk to another.

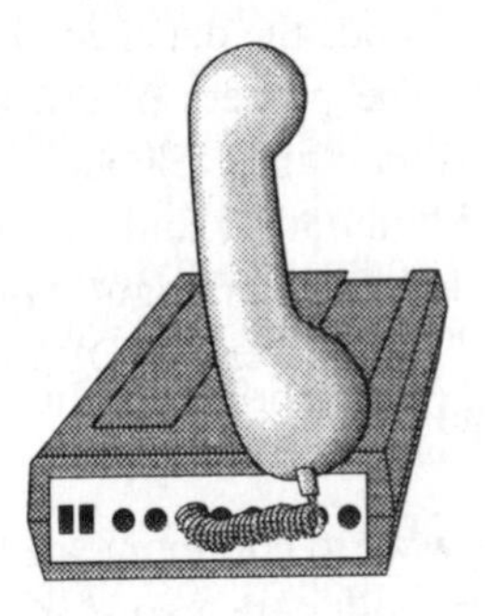

**Figure 2.2** A modem

This device may be inside the computer or sitting next to the computer in a neat little box connected by a cable. There is a slight difficulty when attempting to get one computer to talk to another via the telephone communication channels, since the computer uses a series of electrical pulses to represent characters, whereas with a telephone the electrical signals which represent speech are made up of alternating current waveforms. A modem is used at each end to solve this problem. The

### GLOSSARY OF TERMS 4

**A modem** is a device that enables data to be transmitted between computers, generally over telephone lines, but sometimes on fibre-optic cable or radio frequencies. It enables one computer to talk to another through translating (MOdulating) computer binary signals into telephone analogue signals and back again (DEModulating).

**Facsimile** or **fax** is different from e-mail. Messages, notes, drawings, listings of software and letters which have been prepared using a word processor have to be printed on to paper first. The paper containing the text/drawing is then fed into a fax machine. The machine takes a 'picture' of the text or drawing and transmits the picture to its destination via the telephone line. An ordinary fax machine can communicate with a computer with a fax-modem and vice versa.

computer uses its modem to convert your data into a transmittable form and the receiving computer uses its modem to decode the data back into a form that it can handle. The process of translating the computer digital signals into telephone analogue signals is called MOdulating and the process of translating the telephone analogue signals into computer binary signals is called DEModulating: hence, the name modem.

The computer you want to communicate with must be equipped with a modem that supports the same standard as yours. The nature of the other computer is not necessarily important. Some organizations use modems to connect various computers at different sites. The following are required to use a modem with a telephone network:

- the modem itself;
- a PC or handheld computer;
- the software that allows the modem to be used;
- a telephone socket.

Nearly all modems these days have auto dial and auto receive facilities, and communications software commonly allows you to store your own file of telephone numbers, so that when you wish to transmit to or collect data from a remote computer you simply select the appropriate telephone number and let the computer and modem get on with establishing the connection.

A modem is a valuable addition to any computer system as it can be used for a wide range of communication activities, such as:

- sending messages, letters, documents or data files to other people (*see* e-mail, Section 3.5);
- transferring data to and from bulletin boards (*see* Facts 3);
- transmitting faxes;
- accessing a range of databases;
- downloading shareware and public domain software (*see* Facts 3);
- communicating with other electronic information services, e.g. CompuServe.

A fax-modem is a modem which includes facilities for transmitting data from computers to fax machines and vice versa. With a fax-modem, faxes can be generated using a word processor and sent directly from the computer. Incoming faxes can be received directly into the computer. There are several advantages in this method of sending and receiving faxes.

- Transmitting faxes directly from the computer can save valuable time. You only need to send the fax once. If the distant number is engaged, the computer redials for you until the message gets through.
- Documents can be prepared in advance and scheduled to be sent at a specified date and time.
- Receiving faxes directly into the computer means that the document can be edited before being printed on ordinary paper.
- Perhaps the greatest advantage is that unwanted faxes can be screened out, thus eliminating junk mail, which can be a problem.

The applications of fax-modems in health care or health education include the following.

- Inter-ward or inter-departmental communication. This is instant and cheaper than telephone calls or

## FACTS 3

**Bulletin boards** are electronic 'noticeboards' that make it easy for callers who are interested in a particular topic to leave messages and exchange files.

**Shareware** can be described as a unique marketing strategy. Computer programs are offered free of charge, by some companies, for a trial period ranging from 30 to 90 days. After this period, you are required to pay a registration fee in order to continue using the program. It is quite legal to pass a copy of a shareware program to friends and others. But if they find the program useful, they too are required to become registered users.

**Public domain software** is computer programs that can be freely copied and used.

a trip from Ward A to Ward B.

- Sending and receiving reports/letters to and from a hospital, GP surgery or social services department instantly.
- Using a laptop or notebook computer, primary care workers, such as community psychiatric nurses, community sisters, midwives, health visitors, social workers, general practitioners and so on, can send paperless faxes while on the move.

A radio-modem is a modem that uses radio transmissions to enable fixed and mobile computers to communicate with each other over secure and safe wireless data networks instead of telephone networks. Although wireless data technology was licensed in the UK in 1990, this new network was ready for use only in 1993 and has been attracting users in significant numbers. It is seen as a more flexible and economical mobile communication medium than voice radio and mobile phones. To transmit information using radio modem or wireless data systems the following are required:

- a radio-modem;
- a PC or handheld computer with an RS232 serial port for plugging in the radio-modem;
- appropriate software that allows the modem to be used.

Currently, there are two main public mobile wireless data networks active in the UK. One is operated by Cognito Limited and the other by R A Mobile Data. Wireless data technology can be very useful to health professionals, particularly primary health care workers (*see* 'Wireless data' in Section 3.5).

## 2.4 Scanner

As its name suggests, a scanner is a device used to read words and pictures on a sheet of paper. The pictures might take the form of a photograph, an illustration, a drawing or a logo. The pictures can also be in colour or in black and white. A flatbed scanner looks at a whole page of input, and records and stores the image as a pattern of dots. Once the image is fed into the computer it can be enlarged, reduced or even modified. It can be placed alongside other pictures or text. Using special software known as OCR (optical character recognition), the scanner can read printed or typed documents. Handheld scanners have to be moved manually across the page, which requires a steady hand, whereas flatbed scanners operate along the same lines as a photocopier.

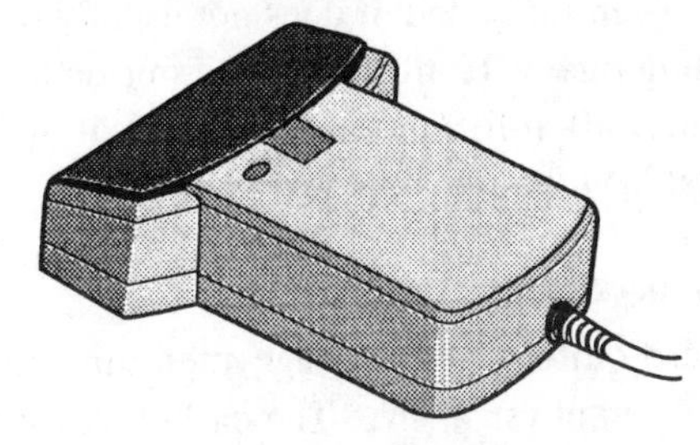

Handheld scanner

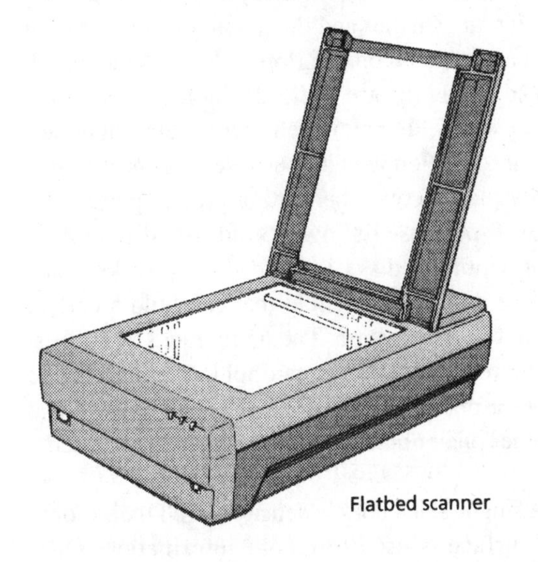

Flatbed scanner

**Figure 2.3** Scanners

An obvious benefit of such a device is that text can be input into the computer quickly without the need to use the keyboard. Once the text is in the computer it can, of course, be edited using a word processing package.

## 2.5 Disks and disk drives

Floppy and hard disks are magnetic media. They provide long-term storage for your data or programs.

Before information can be recorded on to a disk, its surface needs to be mapped in some way by the computer. Unless the surface of the disk has been properly mapped, data cannot be recorded on it. The process of mapping the disk is called **formatting**. A special program is used to format the disk. Once the disk has been formatted, it does not usually require formatting again. If a disk containing data is re-formatted, all information stored on it will be unavailable without disk recovery software.

**Floppy disks or diskettes**

These are quite a new storage medium. Floppy disks vary in physical size. The early types were 8 or 9 inches in diameter. They have been getting smaller and smaller and the amount of information that can be stored on one floppy disk has increased. In use currently are the 5.25 inch and 3.5 inch floppy disks. The 3.5 inch floppy disk does not appear to be floppy at all because it is encased in a sturdy plastic cover, permitting greater portability. Each type has its own kind of disk drive. Information on disks is divided into tracks. Each track is a concentric circle that can hold a certain amount of information. The more tracks a disk has, the more information it can hold. The number of tracks a disk can have depend on its density and whether one or both sides of the disk can be used.

On a single-sided double density (SSDD) disk, only one surface is used to record information. On a double-sided double density (DSDD) disk, both sides are used. A high density (HD) disk can hold approximately twice as much information as a double-sided double density disk or even more.

Disks are sensitive media. They can easily get damaged and work that has taken hours to prepare can be lost. Care of disks is a very important aspect when using computers. To ensure that information stored on your floppy disk is safe, you need to take some simple precautions with regard to handling the disk (*see* 'Care of floppy disk' below).

### GLOSSARY OF TERMS 5

A **floppy disk** is a small flexible medium, usually magnetic, on which information is recorded for future use.

A **hard disk** is an alternative to floppies. It has two or more rigid disks stacked on top of each other in a sealed case. It is much faster, and can store far more data, than a floppy disk.

**Formatting** is the process of preparing a disk so that data can be stored upon it. A special program is used to carry out this process. Once a disk has been formatted it does not normally require formatting again.

**Bytes**. File sizes are measured in bytes. One byte is the amount of space it takes to store a character . A kilobyte (Kb) is 1024 bytes. A megabyte (Mb) is 1024 Kb.

### *FACTS 4*

Six common varieties of disks available

| Type of disks | Space |
|---|---|
| 5.25 inch single-sided double density (SSDD) | 160 and 180 Kb |
| 5.25 inch double-sided double density (DSDD) | 320 and 360 Kb |
| 5.25 inch double-sided high density | 1.2 Mb |
| 3.5 inch double-sided double density (DSDD) | 720 Kb |
| 3.5 inch double-sided high density | 1.44 Mb |
| 3.5 inch double-sided quad density | 2.88 Mb |

**Types of disk drive**

There are different models of disk drives available on the market. By and large one type will accept

5.25 inch disks and the other will accept 3.5 inch disks (Figure 2.4).

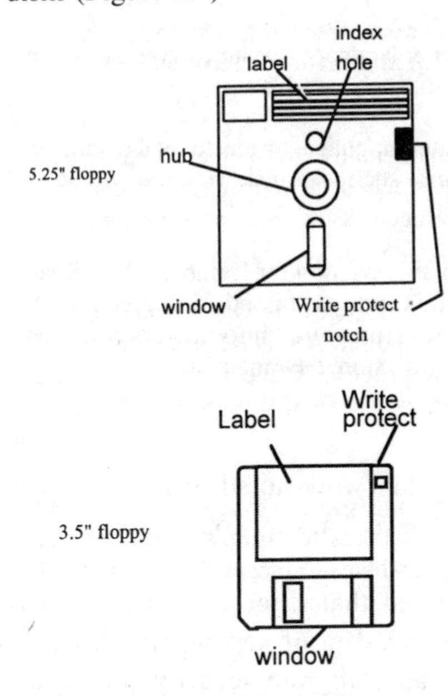


**Figure 2.4** Floppy disks

However, not all types of disks are compatible with all types of drive. As a rule of thumb, always format a disk at a capacity lower than or equal to the capacity of the drive. If the disk and drive are incompatible a 'General failure error' will occur.

In both cases, 5.25 inch and 3.5 inch disks are inserted in the same way. When inserting the disk, make sure the title label on the disk is uppermost. The window should be facing forward to go into the drive first.

Once the disk is in place, some 5.25 inch floppy disk drives have a lever that you need to push down or to the side to prevent the disk jumping out of the drive. For a 3.5 inch disk, push the disk inside the drive until you hear a click. To remove the disk press the button on the front of the drive.

**Anatomy of a floppy disk**

- Label. This indicates what is on the disk. If you are using a 5.25 inch disk, then you should only use a felt tip pen to write on the label, as a pencil or ballpoint pen can damage the disk.
- Write protect notch. Information or data recorded on to disk can be erased intentionally or accidentally. Accidental erasure can be prevented by covering the write-protect notch on a 5.25 inch disk with a self-adhesive tab, or by sliding the built-in tab to leave the notch open on a 3.5 inch disk. When changes need to be made to the data on the disk, the adhesive label can be removed, or the notch closed.
- Index hole. This helps the computer to determine the physical starting point of the data on the disk and its speed of rotation.
- Hub. This helps the drive to secure the disk firmly before it is spun.
- Window. The floppy disk inside the cover can be seen through the window on a 5.25 inch disk, while on the 3.5 inch disk a sliding metal cover exposes part of the disk inside. In either case, when the disk is inserted in the drive, this exposed area is the part of the disk used by the drive to read or write data. Touching the exposed area of the disk at the window might corrupt the information on the disk.

**Care of floppy disks**

Normally information stored on disk will remain intact until you delete it. However, if the disk is damaged, then the information on it may be irretrievable. So take care of your floppy disks and your disks will take care of your information. Here are some 'dos' and 'don'ts'.

Always:

- place the disk back into its envelope;
- keep it in a safe place;
- keep backup copies in different places;
- remove the disk from the disk drive before turning off the computer – failure to do this may result in irreparable damage to the disk.

Do not:

- use magnetized objects near the disk;

- place heavy objects on the disk;
- make erasures near the disk;
- expose the disk to dust or excessive heat or sunlight;
- touch or clean the exposed disk surface;
- fold or bend the disk or use paper clips on it;
- eat, drink or smoke while handling the disk;
- write on it with a ballpoint pen;
- place the disk on top of the monitor or near any magnetic field;
- remove a disk from the drive while the disk drive light is glowing.

## GLOSSARY OF TERMS 6

**Write**, in computer language, means to save data on to a storage medium, such as a disk.

**Read**, in computer language, means to load data from a storage medium, such as a disk, into the computer memory (RAM).

**CD-ROM** is an abbreviation for Compact Disk-Read Only Memory. It is one type of optical storage media. The user can only retrieve the information stored on this type of disk, not store new material.

### The hard disk

The hard disk, as its name suggests, is not flexible. It can be an integral part of a computer. Although hard disks use a different type of disk drive from floppies, both hard and floppy disks function in basically the same way. Magnetic heads **read** information from the disk into the computer's memory or **write** data from the computer's memory on to the surface of the disk.

The heads of the hard disk do not come into contact with the disk surface but float above it on a cushion of air. Thus hard disks do not suffer as much wear as floppies. Heads must be 'parked', i.e. dismounted, when the computer is not in use. Modern computers do this automatically when the machine is switched off.

Storage space on a hard disk ranges from 5 to over 1000 Mb and the speed of data storage and retrieval is significantly faster than the corresponding speed of floppy disk operation. As an example, floppy disks typically rotate at between 200 and 360 r.p.m. but hard disks rotate in the region of 3600 r.p.m. A hard disk is housed inside the computer casing. There now exist exchangeable hard disks which are inserted in a disk drive in a similar way to a floppy disk.

### Protecting information

For extra security of data against accidental loss or damage, all important work stored on disks – floppy or hard – should have 'backup' copies.

It is recommended that three copies of a disk containing important data are kept in three different places. This is an elaborate security procedure which, unfortunately, often tends to be taken seriously only after a bitter experience involving loss of data or floppy disk corruption. In this case, it really is better to be safe than sorry.

## 2.6 Optical disks

Another storage medium which has entered the market is the optical disk. Optical technology is similar in principle to the compact disk (CD) used for audio recording. Three basic types of optical disk are in existence: CD-ROM, WORM and magneto-optical.

### CD-ROM

This is an acronym for Compact Disk-Read Only Memory. As a user, you cannot store your own information on a CD-ROM. All information contained on this type of disk is implanted at manufacture, in the same way that music is recorded on a CD. This type of disk is already popular with libraries as each one can hold a vast amount of text. CD-ROMs can store pictures as well as text, and may soon become a common medium for storing information in clinical settings.

**WORM**

This is an acronym for Write Once Read Many times. This is a more advanced medium than CD-ROM. With this storage medium you, as the user, can enter your own data. However, these data can never be erased. A WORM device is an alloy disk, covered on both sides by plastic. A laser burns holes in the plastic, and these burnt pits represent the data. To read the data, a low powered laser is passed over the disk and the reflected light is detected.

**Magneto-optical**

The magneto-optical disk is a recent development. These disks comprise a magnetized recording medium sandwiched between two plastic disks. The content of the disk can be altered magnetically at high temperatures. The area to be altered is heated by a laser, and its magnetic charge is reversed by this process. The main advantage of optical disks over other storage media is that large amounts of data can be stored on one disk.

## GLOSSARY OF TERMS 7

**WORM** is an acronym for Write Once Read Many times. This is like the CD-ROM except that the user can enter his or her own data, but only once.

**Magneto-optical** is a storage medium. Unlike CD-ROM or WORM, the content of the disk can be altered.

## *FACTS 5*

IBM (International Business Machine) or IBM compatible machines, Apple Macintosh, Acorn 3000, Amiga and Atari ST are a few computer systems on the market. A program written for IBM machines will not work on Apple, Acorn or Atari computers without conversion.

A disk prepared for use with IBM or IBM compatible machines or with one kind of operating system cannot be used with another (except with the use of special programs).

## Suggested Assignments

AIM — To explore the usefulness of various input and output devices for personal and professional use.

ACTIVITY 1 — Nowadays most hospital and college libraries store bibliographic information on CD-ROM. Carry out a literature search on the application of computers in nursing or on any other topic of your choice using CD-ROM. Enlist the help of the librarian as appropriate. (For a short guide see Appendix 9.)

ACTIVITY 2 — Consider the benefits of using optical disks in clinical settings for the storage and retrieval of information about patients/clients and staff.

ACTIVITY 3 — Find out if your college or place of work has a scanner. If not, perhaps you could try a nearby library. Enlisting the help of a knowledgeable person, scan a piece of text and graphics using a flatbed or handheld scanner. Now, think how health care workers can make use of such a piece of equipment.

ACTIVITY 4 — A modem can be used for a range of communication activities. Using information given in this book and from your reading of available material and personal experience, list as many activities as you can that can be performed using a modem.

ACTIVITY 5 A modem is an invaluable addition to a computer set-up in health care settings. But it also mean that the computer is no longer a closed system. Consider the possible dangers associated with such a system and think of ways of minimizing risks.

## Endnote

Now that you have completed this unit, you should be able to:

- list four devices that can be connected to a computer;
- differentiate between a fax and a modem;
- explain what you understand by the term formatting;
- explain the purpose of formatting a disk;
- list 14 precautions that you should take when handling a floppy disk;
  compare and contrast the print quality of various types of printers;
- appraise the use of various input and output devices in health care settings.

# Self-Assessment Test for Unit 3

## Instructions

Answer the following questions. Decide how confident you feel about each of your answers and mark your score in the column provided or on a piece of paper. The weighting for each question is shown in the right-hand column. When you have answered all the questions, add up your marks. Then look at the scoreometer to determine your rating

| No. | Question | Expected Score | Actual Score |
|---|---|---|---|
| 1 | List five functions of a computer. *(1 mark each)* | 5 | |
| 2 | List two possible uses of a word processor in clinical settings. *(1 mark each)* | 2 | |
| 3 | What are its advantages over a typewriter? *(4 marks)* | 4 | |
| 4 | What is a database application program? | 4 | |
| 5 | State two advantages and two disadvantages of such a system in the ward situation. *(1 mark each)* | 4 | |
| 6 | List four possible uses for a spreadsheet in clinical settings. *(1 mark each)* | 4 | |
| 7 | What do you understand by e-mail? | 1 | |
| 8 | (a) How can e-mail be used by practitioners to enhance care? *(1 mark)*<br>(b) List two advantages and two disadvantages of such a system. *(1 mark each)* | 5 | |
| 9 | What is the meaning of LAN and WAN and how do they differ? | 3 | |
| 10 | Name one statistical package that can be used to analyse nursing data. | 1 | |
| 11 | (a) What is an expert system? *(1 mark)*<br>(b) How can expert systems be used in clinical areas? *(2 marks)* | 3 | |
| | **Total score** | **36** | |

## Scoreometer

**33 to 36** You can skip this unit if you are absolutely confident with your answers.
**18 to 32** You should at least survey this unit.
**9 to 17** You would be well advised to read relevant sub-sections of this unit.
**0 to 8** You would benefit from reading the whole unit.

# UNIT 3
# What tasks can the computer do?

If properly instructed the computer can perform very sophisticated functions as described in the next few pages more quickly than a human being ever can. Its strength lies in the hands of computer literate users.

## 3.1 Word processing

The basic uses for a word processor are similar to those of a typewriter – but it can perform a broader range of tasks with much greater speed, flexibility and convenience. The concept is simple. Instead of the words appearing on a sheet of paper as you type, they appear on the computer screen – the monitor discussed in Unit 1. The whole document is held in the computer's memory and can be altered on screen, where all necessary corrections and changes can be made and viewed before printing. If your word processing software also contains a **spell checker** you will be able to run a simple program which will check that every word in your document is spelt correctly.

Some advanced word processing packages provide facilities such as a **grammar checker**, word counts, columns, indexing, table contents, graphics and so on.

Should additional changes need to be made, the whole document does not need to be retyped (or 'rekeyed') but simply called back to the screen, corrected and reprinted. Word processing (WP) software will go a long way towards making your document look a lot more professional. If you want to send the same letter to several addresses, it does not have to be rekeyed every time but can simply be stored on a disk. Depending on the type of printer you use, a good word processor can help make someone new to typing look like a professional. If you have to do all the typing yourself and don't know where to start, several typing tutor programs are available to help you. A word processor is invaluable for anyone who does a lot of writing. Health professionals can use it for:

- writing general correspondence and memos;
- recording patients' or clients' notes and reports;
- developing instruments, such as questionnaires for research;
- analysing qualitative data;

### GLOSSARY OF TERMS 8

A **word processor** can be thought of as similar to a typewriter. To use it text must be typed in from the keyboard. However, it offers several advantages over the traditional typewriter.

A **spell checker** is a computer program which allows the user to check that every word in a document is spelt correctly. Only the more expensive word processing packages have this facility.

A **grammar checker** is a computer program which allows the user to check grammatical errors. The program will display suggestions, which you can ignore if you choose to.

### *FACTS 6*

Word™, WordPerfect™ and Ami Pro™ are three of the most sophisticated and popular word processing packages available currently.

## GLOSSARY OF TERMS 9

**WYSIWYG** is an acronym for What You See Is What You Get. The way the document appears on the screen display closely resembles the way it will appear on paper when it is printed. An invaluable feature of a good word processing package.

**Desktop** is a term used to refer to a computer that is usually placed somewhere on a desk

A **desktop publishing** application, also referred to as DTP, is a sophisticated word processor. It offers greater control over the finished document

## *FACTS 7*

Windows (written with a capital W) is the name of a product produced by the US company Microsoft, while windows (written with a lowercase w) refers to frame areas of the computer screen. The product Windows can be described as a collection of programs written for personal computers. (See Unit 8 for more information.)

- preparing transparencies and handouts;
- writing articles, reports and books for publication;
- writing academic assignments, such as essays, projects and dissertations.

The list is endless. Using an electric or manual typewriter, how fast can you type? Whatever your speed, invariably you will slow down whenever you have to stop and correct your errors. One of the good things about word processing is that correcting typing errors has never been easier.

All word processing packages make use of the familiar 'QWERTY' keyboard. Word processing packages for use in a Windows environment, include facilities for using a mouse. Voice-activated word processors are not widely available yet.

Although there are several types of word processing packages, the principles of use are generally the same. As with everything else, a period of training is necessary in order to understand fully the strength and pitfalls of the word processor being used. A brief summary of the benefits of word processing over typing using a traditional manual or electric typewriter is given in Table 3.1.

As you might expect there are also some disadvantages. The user has to face a screen for a long period of time. This could lead to health problems (*see* Section 6.4).

During the learning stage paper wastage may become a concern. Unless you are using a **WYSIWYG** system (What You See Is What You Get), it may not be possible to see what the document will look like before it is printed. This may be problematic when different fonts and facilities, such as bold, underscoring or italics, are used. Learning to use all the facilities included in a word processing package takes time and practice. This powerful application tool is only as good as its user.

## 3.2 Desktop publishing

**Desktop publishing**, or DTP as it is called, is an even more sophisticated form of word processing. While WP gives the user control over the text input, DTP offers the user greater control over the final look of the document as well as high quality presentations. This includes the style and size of typeface ('font') used as well as the number of columns on a page. Text prepared on your word processor can be used with your DTP program to save any rekeying. Some DTP programs enable the user to create his or her own pictures, graphs and drawings on screen.

There are many DTP programs available, which range from simple enhanced word processors to full page make-up programs used to design and lay out magazines. DTPs are becoming increasingly user friendly. Anyone can learn how to use such programs without difficulty.

Like any other organization, hospitals, daycare

centres, GP surgeries, colleges of nursing and so on produce a wide range of documents, such as annual reports, newsletters, compliment slips, letterheads and so on. Sometimes outside typesetters are engaged for this task. Ward or departmental staff very often produce hand-written fly sheets and notices. All these can be produced in-house quickly with a high finish by the use of a computer and laser printer.

**FACTS 8**

**Ventura™, Pagemaker™ and MS Publisher for Windows™ are three well known DTP packages.**

| | Word processor | Manual or electric typewriter |
|---|---|---|
| **Editing** | You can correct and change a document before producing it on paper.<br>Once text has been entered it is easy to reformat it with different line widths or to reset margins and page lengths.<br>Revisions of text can be achieved with little effort. | Mistakes have to be corrected using erasers, leaving behind unsightly marks.<br>The entire document will need to be retyped if a different specification is required.<br>Large revision of text is laborious and can only be achieved by retyping the entire document. |
| **Storage** | Letters and documents can be stored on disk or tape in a fraction of the space needed for conventional files, and can often be retrieved more quickly. | Letters and documents have to be stored in cabinets, taking up a lot of space, and, even with a good classification system, can be difficult and time-consuming to retrieve. |
| **Standard letters** | Standard letters can be reproduced quickly with new names and addresses. | Standard letters have to be typed and addressed individually. |
| **Mail shots** | Using one standard letter, it is possible to add personal addresses for many different people. The advantage is that everyone seems to have been sent an original letter and will treat it as such. | Personal addresses have to be added individually after the standard letter has been typed. This means more time is required to do the task. |
| **Printing** | The availability of special print facilities, such as bold, italics, foreign characters, large/extra large, shadowed characters and so on, means that styling a document can be achieved with ease. | Even on modern electric (or even some electronic) typewriters, print facilities are limited and require constant stopping and changing of daisywheels. With manual typewriters the print facility is limited to one type style. |
| **Spelling** | Generally a spell checker is available to check the entire document for errors and to permit changes to be made. | Spelling mistakes often mean that the document has to be retyped. |
| **Thesaurus** | The availability of a thesaurus allows for a quick choice of words. You can even have your own personal dictionary. | A thesaurus can be handy if you can find one when needed. Without it you will have to struggle. |
| **Grammar** | The document can be checked for proper use of grammar. | Grammatical mistakes could mean that the document or part of it has to be retyped. |
| **Size** | Word processors frequently have a word counter built into them, which allows you accurately to count the number of words in a document quickly. | Words have to be counted manually. In a document of 10,000 words or more this can be very time-consuming. |
| **Sorting** | Selected paragraphs can be arranged alphabetically or numerically with ease. | Reordering paragraphs means retyping the document. |
| **Electronic mail** | In order to prepare material for transmission, you need to use a word processor and a computer linked to the telephone system to send documents through the telephone system. (This is different from using a facsimile (fax) machine, which takes a 'picture' of text and transmits the picture to its destination.) | Although it is possible to prepare a document to send as a fax, direct transmission through an electronic mail system is not possible. |

**Table 3.1** A comparison of word processors and traditional manual or electric typewriters

## 3.3 Databases

**Database** work is far more sophisticated than a card index system. A database can be described as a sophisticated electronic filing cabinet capable of storing and sorting large amounts of data in an organized manner. Unlike a metal filing cabinet with lots of paper files in it, all the information in a database is saved on disk(s).

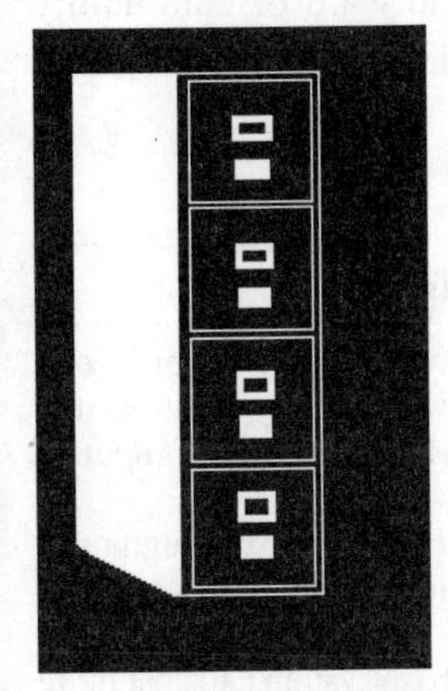

**Figure 3.1** One database can replace several manual filing cabinets. Think of the space that is saved

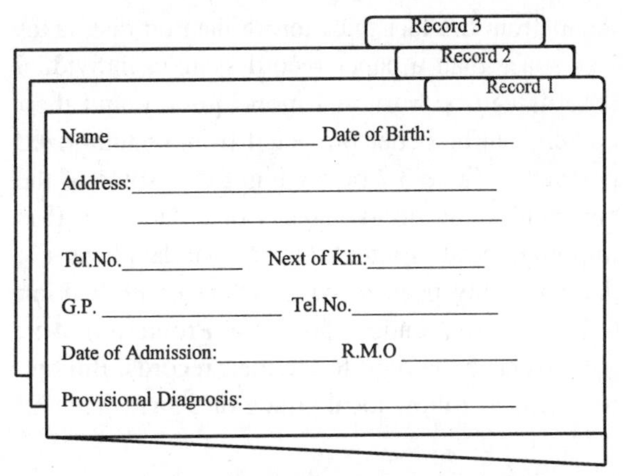


**Figure 3.2** A database file showing three records. Each record has nine fields: Name, Date of birth, Address, Tel. no., Next of kin, GP, Date of admission, RMO and Provisional diagnosis

A database has 'files'. Each **file** is made up of 'records' and each record contains 'fields'. A **field** would contain a relevant piece of information, such as the name of the person or organization. In Figure 3.2 each **record** has ten fields. How many records you have in a file and how many fields you have in each record will depend on the information you want to keep and the database package you are using.

A variety of information can be held on files on magnetic disk, which can then be quickly accessed at any time. Such information (data) may include clients' or patients' names and their personal details, treatment records, nursing care plans and so on.

The data in the database can be deleted or amended as required. New data can be added. By giving your database a simple command you can search for similar entries such as all patients or clients who have had surgery in the past six months or have been discharged under the care of a particular community nurse or midwife.

Information in the database, such as the names and addresses of clients or patients, can be sorted as desired and printed on paper. Of course, a database concerned with hospital patients will need updating when patients are discharged or admitted. Unless the database is updated regularly its value will be drastically reduced.

### GLOSSARY OF TERMS 10

**Data** are raw facts and figures.

A **database** can be described as a sophisticated electronic filing cabinet capable of sorting data in an organized manner. The data can be accessed quickly as desired.

A **file** is a collection of related information, like the contents of a file folder in a desk drawer.

**Record.** In the context of a database each card is called a record.

**Field.** In the context of a database each title or subtitle on a record is referred to as a field (the term also refers to an area of a screen that is designated to hold a specified piece of information).

Apart from the fact that storing data on disk takes less space than a paper record system, individual records can be retrieved more quickly and their content can be better protected from unauthorized personnel. Table 3.2 below highlights some of the advantages and disadvantages of a database. It is important not to forget that personal data kept in a database may need to be registered (*see* Section 6.2). Equally, under the Data Protection Act, patients have the right to see their records. But one will need to follow local policy on how, when and who should give information and with what interpretative assistance. The ward or community manager should be aware of the local process.

### FACTS 9

**Corel Draw™**, **Paintbrush™** and **Aldus Freehand™** are three graphic programs on the market.

**Paradox™**, **FoxPro™**, **DataEase™** and **dBase IV™** are some of the commercial database packages currently available.

| Advantages | Disadvantages |
|---|---|
| • **No duplication**. There is less duplication of data than with a conventional filing system. Data can be used for many purposes but only need to be input and stored once. For example, the code number, name and address of each patient/client is input and stored once, instead of several times (as tends to happen with manual systems – especially when patients are moved around from one ward to another or discharged and readmitted). | • **Centralization**. With single entry input one department in the hospital or community health centre must accept responsibility for the accuracy of input. |
| • **Integration**. Several departments or community centres can share data, not just the individual ward, unit or health centre. | • **Time**. Setting up a database takes time, although once it is set up it will serve for a long time. |
| • **Input**. Multiple files containing the same data can be updated quickly with single input from one department. Thus, the overall time taken for such administrative activities is drastically reduced. | • **Cost**. A good electronic database system can cost more than a conventional system. |
| • **Speed**. Quick access to information. There is no need to wait for the patient's notes to arrive. As soon as you know a patient is being transferred to your ward you can quiz the database for relevant information about him or her. | • **Expertise**. Specially trained staff are required to manage the system effectively. |
| • **Space**. A variety of information can be stored on disks, which require less space than filing cabinets that are old and sometimes poorly maintained. | • **Crash**. When the system is down, access to all information can be a problem. |
| • **Consistency**. All data are stored in a particular format. | • **Security and privacy**. Preventing data from being altered by unauthorized people (i.e. data security) and preserving the confidentiality of the data (i.e. data privacy) can be a problem. A partial solution to the problem involves control of terminal access, user identification and restrictions to access by certain users to certain programs or certain parts of the database (*see* Section 6.1). |
| • **Flexibility**. Information in a database can be analysed and presented in new ways. | • **Corruption**. Since there is only one set of data, data corruption can be severe and costly. |

**Table 3.2** Some advantages and disadvantages of a database

## 3.4 Spreadsheets (for financial control, planning, research)

A computer can be a significant boon in streamlining finances and giving greater control over a business. As in any business, nurses and health care professionals need to handle numerical data. For instance, you may need to:

- make financial forecasts;
- monitor stocks of drugs;
- order dressings and stationery;
- prepare a staff rota or record holidays.

Nursing lecturers also need to handle numeric and alphanumeric tasks, such as:

- scheduling student placements;
- analysing examination results;
- tabulating and calculating teaching hours.

There are a number of software application programs to help in these cases, the spreadsheet being the most basic type.

A spreadsheet can be viewed as an electronic ledger with horizontal rows and vertical columns. At their points of intersection pigeon-holes are formed, usually called cells. Words, figures and formulae can all be added to these cells (Figure 3.3).

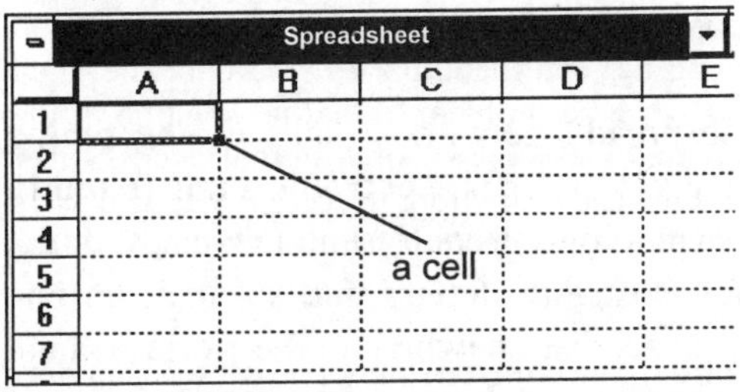

**Figure 3.3** A spreadsheet

The beauty of a spreadsheet is in how these figures can be manipulated. Instead of you adding up the figures in your head, the spreadsheet software will do it for you, producing a series of totalled figures – across a row, or down a column – at the touch of a button.

### GLOSSARY OF TERMS 11

A **document** is a piece of work with a specific name, produced on a computer, which if stored can be retrieved immediately or at a later time.

A **spreadsheet** is an electronic sheet with horizontal rows and vertical columns forming cells at each point of intersection. Words, figures and formulae can all be added to the cells and calculations can be performed with the minimum of effort.

### *FACTS 10*

**Quattro Pro™, Lotus 123™** and **Excel™** are among the leading spreadsheet packages currently available.

The formulae can be very simple. For example, telling the spreadsheet to: 'add all the items in rows 1 to 7 of column B and print the total in this cell' would be as simple as writing the words 'SUM(B1..B7)' in the cell where you want the total to appear. The most common use of a spreadsheet is for budgeting and speculating about your departmental finances. This is known as asking 'what if?' questions: you can change, perhaps, the cost of an item and see just what its full implications would be. The spreadsheet software also contains a variety of financial, mathematical and statistical formulae to help you. The computer spreadsheet is the perfect electronic tool or application program for handling some of the dreary tasks that take hours to do, i.e. any information that can be represented as columns and rows. It is easier to use an electronic spreadsheet than to perform calculations manually and any manual stock control system can be computerized. Some packages are so sophisticated that the computer will take note of items used and then reorder them automatically.

## 3.5 Communication networks

In big organizations where several computers may be required, there is little point in installing stand-alone systems. Apart from being costly, stand-alone computer systems usually function independently from one another and, since each computer system is working in isolation from the others, there is no sharing of resources. Programs installed on one computer are not available to another and data entered on one system can normally only be accessed from that system. Furthermore the opportunity to improve communication is being denied. To make all programs and data from one system accessible to other users regardless of the physical location of the resource, and to enable messages to be sent from one terminal to another, all the individual systems must be connected together to form a network. If a system of interconnected computers and other devices is spread over a small area, typically within a few hundred yards and linked by cables, it is called a **local area network (LAN)**.

In contrast, a **wide area network (WAN)**, or **long haul network (LHN)** is a network spread over a wide geographical area and typically sends data over telecommunications links. Such a network can provide a powerful medium for communication between users separated by quite a distance. For instance, two or more users, each living in different towns or even in different countries, could write a report or a book together.

When one author makes a change to the document, which is kept on-line, the others can see the change immediately, instead of waiting several days for a letter. Such speed makes cooperation among far-flung groups of people easy where it was once impossible. The application of such a system in clinical or educational settings can enhance interpersonal communication and reduce – or even eliminate – any duplication of records kept.

When a client is transferred from one ward to another, from one hospital to another, or even from hospital to after-care in the community, there is no need to wait impatiently for the old case notes to arrive or to waste time collecting the same information over and over again.

## GLOSSARY OF TERMS 12

**Network** is a general term used to describe the connection of compatible computers.

**LAN** refers to a system of interconnected PCs and other devices over a small area, typically within a few hundred yards, linked directly by cables. It is an abbreviation for local area network.

**WAN** refers to a network of computers located far afield. It is an abbreviation for wide area network.

**Long haul network** is an alternative term for WAN.

**Electronic mail** or **e-mail** is a relatively new concept in human communications. It allows people to send each other information, messages, notes, drawings, software and letters immediately without putting them to paper.

The availability of a (public) WAN makes many new applications feasible. For example, remote databases can be accessed at the touch of a button. A hospital or educational establishment that has produced a new technique for evaluating standards of care may allow other institutions to log in over the network and run the program to see how useful the technique is.

A widespread network that is becoming increasingly popular is **electronic mail (e-mail)**. This system allows users to send messages, notes, drawings, software, letters and so on from one terminal to another anywhere in the world without putting pen to paper. It is a relatively new concept in human communication. Words and symbols are created using the computer and then sent to a recipient via the telephone line using a modem.

E-mail is effectively an electronic post office. It is immediate. There is no need to rely on the traditional postal system to deliver important messages. At the other end of the line the messages wait until the recipient checks whether any messages have been received. If the recipient happens to be on-line he or she can read your message almost instantly, without having to wait for the postman to deliver it. Messages can be left in someone's e-mail box at any time of day or night.

Unlike with ordinary post, the address is not a fixed location like a house, but an individual. The message is stored in a central computer and thousands of other users have their mailboxes on the same computer system. Therefore the individual can receive and send e-mail from anywhere in Britain or abroad. The word 'mail' implies a personal message and each user has a unique identification code which ensures that users only get the messages intended for them. Table 3.3 shows some of the advantages and disadvantages of e-mail.

## FACTS 11

**The basic requirement for e-mail is a modem, a computer fitted with a special board, communications software and a telephone line.**

**National systems offer more facilities to users and are therefore more expensive. There is usually an initial joining fee and then a monthly bill for connection as well as peak hour telephone charges.**

| Advantages | Disadvantages |
|---|---|
| **Cost.** The cost of producing printed copies of messages/letters/documents is transferred to the recipient, which saves the sender a lot of printing or photocopying. It is claimed that communication costs can be reduced by nine-tenths. | **Junk-mail.** Unwanted mail can consume valuable time and it will also cost money to get rid of them. |
| **Speed.** As soon as the message is sent it is ready for the recipient to read. | **Hasty responses.** The facility to respond immediately can encourage hasty, thoughtless replies. |
| **No blackholes.** Messages do not get lost. It is even possible to have an automatic acknowledgement that your message has been received. | **Unintentional deletion.** Important mail can be deleted by mistake. Extra care should make this less of a problem. |
| **Flexible timing.** Messages can be sent at any time of day or night and on any day of the week, including holidays. | **Ill-prepared mail.** Inaccurate headings on mail received could waste your time. |
| **Flexible location.** Messages can be sent to or received from someone anywhere in the world. All that is needed is a suitable terminal. | **Garbage.** Mail may be corrupted if the line being used is too noisy. |
| **Accessibility.** E-mail systems are always open. There is no need for multiple phone calls, or to leave a message (which may not be passed on) with a third party because the person you want is not available. | **Forbidden correspondence.** Invoices and writs, for example, cannot be sent by e-mail. |
| **Control.** A message can be sent and its delivery can be purposely delayed. This is useful in preparing documents well in advance but delaying their distribution until a later date. | **Deception.** The ability to delay the delivery of a message can encourage trickery and make it difficult for the receiver to establish the exact date the message was written. |
| **Multiple copies.** A letter or document can be sent to several people concurrently, saving money and valuable time on photocopies and addressing individual envelopes. It takes 25 seconds to send an A4 sheet and 10 minutes to send a 10,000 word document. | **Duplication.** Letters or documents may have to be duplicated for those who cannot receive them by electronic means. |
| **Choice of storage.** Messages/documents received can be kept on disk or printed on paper. You can even make alterations to the received document before printing it. | **Unwanted cost.** Storing received mail can be costly. |
| **Confidentiality.** Thanks to the clever use of passwords, only the addressee can read the message. If a box is shared, private messages can be sent which require an extra password to be typed before they can be read. This password can be arranged in advance with the person concerned. | **Security.** This can be a problem. The chances of a whiz-kid breaking into your mail box is always there, although frequent changing of passwords could minimize this risk. |

**Table 3.3** Some advantages and disadvantages of electronic mail

Like anything else, e-mail will not meet all our needs. Equally there are as many disadvantages of e-mail as there are advantages (*see* Table 3.3). However, it can be argued that the advantages by far outweigh the disadvantages. E-mail can be a very useful facility for nurse tutors, nursing students and practitioners alike.

- Nursing students can increase their range of communication skills and extend their use of language by drafting and sending messages to foreign nursing students, and can compare their ideas with other students from other colleges.
- Nursing tutors and lecturers can exchange ideas, information and materials with a wide range of tutors in other colleges or can receive data from other helpful agencies quickly and easily.
- Practitioners can establish contacts with specialists in the same field to obtain news about new approaches in other hospitals and to see if they are worth adopting, or leave messages to colleagues working on other wards or community centres.
- Community psychiatric nurses or health visitors can contact local social workers about a particular family case. They can also send files and data 'back to base' from a portable or notebook computer, while on the move.

**Wireless data transmission** is yet another system which allows users to send written messages from one computer to another without putting pen to paper. With this system, words are created using fixed or mobile computers and then sent to a recipient via a wireless link using a radio-modem. To transmit information using wireless data one follows four easy steps:

- plug a radio-modem into a PC or handheld computer;
- key in the message or data;
- add the network address;
- press the send button.

The information reaches the addressee's computer via a local radio-based station. There is one essential difference between the wireless data system and e-mail or fax-modem systems. While the last two use telephone lines to transmit information from one computer to another, wireless data systems replace the telephone links by wireless links. Since there is no need to be near a telephone socket to connect the modem when transmitting messages, this is a more flexible system. Hamilton (1993) suggests that, when sending messages to one or more members of a group – e.g. a primary health care team who are out and about – it is cheaper to use a wireless data system than 'voice' wireless systems or even mobile phones. Such a system certainly has benefits to health professionals. Hamilton identifies several of them, which have been summarized in Table 3.4.

## GLOSSARY OF TERMS 13

A **gateway** is an interface, perhaps between networks, perhaps between a network and a major computer system, and usually involves both hardware and software.

**TTNS (The Times Network Systems)** provides a multi-faceted communications and information service through the medium of information technology. It is a service to education as a whole.

**JANET (Joint Academic Network)** is a government-funded computer network. It is designed to support UK academic and research communities, by providing access to other institution facilities (e.g. library catalogues, research banks, on-line conferences), and by allowing communication with members of those institutions via e-mail.

Access to a central computer offers many more facilities. For example, a central computer can be linked in to the telex service, thereby allowing users to send and receive messages on telex. It also gives access to various **electronic bulletin board** services, such as Telecom Gold and Campus 2000. The Telecom Gold bulletin board, for example, can be accessed at the > prompt by entering NOTICEBD. It includes a range of categories, including one for lonely hearts. Another major area of network use is gateways to databases providing specialized information services, such as the **Joint Academic Network (JANET)** for library reservation, catalogues and so on and **The Times Network System (TTNS).**

The English National Board database on TTNS can be accessed via menus and information can be downloaded for reference or for educational purposes. In addition, the literature database can be searched for occurrences of particular references.

In some hospitals, patient information is communicated around the hospital using a computer network which links all major departments into a common database of patient information. Using a ward terminal, information can be sent to and received from all patient-care areas.

With an automated communication system nurses no longer have to spend time writing requests or answering the phone for results from the Pathology

| Some of the useful facilities provided by wireless data | Corresponding benefits of using a wireless data system |
|---|---|
| **One-way messaging.** Within a few seconds of sending a message, you get a notification of the receipt of your message on your computer screen. | A message can be sent to one or several members of a group, such as a primary health care team, who may be on the move, and you will know that they have received it.<br>It is a cost-effective way of getting information to one or more individuals quickly.<br>Unlike with conventional message paging, there is :<br>• no need to telephone a pager company and dictate the message;<br>• an acknowledgement that the message has been received or stored;<br>• a copy of the message on the computer. |
| **Two-way messaging.** Individuals can exchange messages at a distance. | A cheaper way of communicating than using the mobile phone.<br>No engaged telephone numbers, hence no time wasting.<br>Your message gets through immediately but the receiver can respond when it is convenient. |
| **Facsimile transmission.** A message can be typed on the computer and sent to a distant fax number in seconds. | No need to worry if the distant telephone number is engaged. The system will redial and get your message through.<br>You do not need a fax machine yourself to communicate with one.<br>Paperless faxes can be sent from anywhere, such as from the patient's home, a clinic or a car. |
| **Access to distant computers.** You can view and add to information on distant computers provided you have the right password and PIN number. | Primary health care workers, such as GPs, community psychiatric nurses, community sisters, midwives, social workers, physiotherapists and occupational therapists, can access, view and update the records of their patients/clients or view a hospital poisons information service at a distant. |
| **Remote telemetry.** With an ultra-sound transducer monitor connected to a portable computer, the development of unborn children in pregnant mothers can be safely monitored in the community. | Using the graphical read-outs on uterine activity, maternal blood pressure, foetal heart rate and foetal body movements displayed on the computer screen, midwives can safely monitor the development of unborn children during their domiciliary visits, thus reducing unnecessary hospital visits to see consultants.<br>Using the two-way messaging facility, midwives can seek and obtain expert help on abnormal readings within minutes and arrange for hospital admissions if need be. |

**Table 3.4** Some facilities and benefits of wireless data systems (adapted from an article by Hamilton, 1993)

or X-ray departments. Using the computer network as a sophisticated communication system may also reduce the amount of travelling done, thus saving energy, time and money – three valuable resources.

Unfortunately, in the majority of hospitals a fragmented computer system is currently in operation. Various departments have stand-alone systems. Information is printed and transferred manually to other departments. Obviously such a system is not as fast and efficient as a network. It does not allow the free flow of information. In fact, this is a clear example of the underuse of a powerful and expensive resource.

Looking on the bright side, quite a few computerized nursing information systems are up and running in the United Kingdom, and many more are in the pipeline. The Devon and Exeter System and the Ninewells System in Dundee are quoted by Koch and Rankin (1987) as the most well-known. They report that the Ninewells System has demonstrated the benefits of producing a clear, concise nursing-care plan, from which future developments could allow a nursing workload index to be derived. There is evidence that the wide area network between different health disciplines is growing. Such a communication system, The Times Network System, is already in existence in the areas of nursing and midwifery education.

## 3.6 Statistics

Research is an area that is being taken more seriously in both clinical settings and nursing education. To facilitate analysis of data, various statistical packages are available. These include SPSS (Statistical Packages for the Social Sciences), SAS (Statistical Analysis System), BMCP (Biomedical Computer Programs) and Minitab. These statistical packages have been developed for the microcomputer as well as the **mainframe** to make data analysis less time-consuming. The mathematical formulae are built into the program (for more information see Unit 10).

## 3.7 Expert systems

The area of **expert systems** is presently developing rapidly. An expert system is a computer program. It enables a 'knowledge engineer' or analyst to build a 'knowledge base' of information elicited from an expert (or experts) in a specific domain. The knowledge of an expert or experts is fed into a computer using an expert system **'shell'**. The shell is simply the package that holds and manipulates the knowledge base. In theory an expert system should provide a rapid answer to a particular problem, or might be able to examine information so as to pinpoint any problem and its solution. Put another way, you type in certain facts and the program uses its information on file to produce a decision about something for which an expert would normally be required. Doctors can use an expert medical system to arrive at a medical diagnosis while nurses can use an expert nursing system to arrive at a nursing diagnosis.

Quite a few expert system shells for microcomputers are in existence. The Crystal expert system shell is particularly noteworthy in that it has been used by the Departments of Health and Social

### GLOSSARY OF TERMS 14

A **mainframe** is a large computer with a large amount of memory which has the ability to serve several users simultaneously.

An **expert system** is a computer program which possesses knowledge rather than figures and words. The program must use logical reasoning procedures, allowing problems to be solved

A **shell** is a computer program that holds and manipulates the data constituting the knowledge base.

Security to produce an expert system that is claimed to identify district health authority performance problems based on performance indicator data.

There are obvious benefits to expert systems. As Eaton (1991) points out, an expert system can:

- **improve productivity** – readily available knowledge can help to get the job done quickly;
- **preserve knowledge** – in the absence of a particular expert, his or her knowledge can still be available for use if it has been acquired and appropriately packaged into a usable expert system;
- **improve understanding and learning** – expert systems can aid understanding of how an expert goes about solving a problem.

There are four main parts to an expert system.

- **The knowledge base**. This is made up of facts (such as 'tinea is a fungal infection of the skin') and rules (such as 'tinea is contagious, avoid contact').
- **The knowledge acquisition program**. This is a program which enables the expert system to learn new facts and rules.
- **The control program/inference engine**. This interprets the input into the program, and in the light of the facts and rules stored with the knowledge base, arrives at an answer or a diagnosis.
- **The user interface**. This is perhaps the most important part of the expert system. It is the means by which the expert system communicates with the user. It can request additional information from the user before offering a reply/diagnosis.

The expert system may be designed to accept enquiries in something very close to everyday English.

Such a system can improve nursing practice by its ability to enhance the decision-making process and influence planning and implementation of nursing care. While this powerful tool can aid the nurse with her decision-making, it cannot and should not be viewed as a substitute for the nurse–patient relationship and contact. The computer is a means of improving the quantity and quality of nursing care and as such is just a helpful friend.

## FACTS 12

**Decision Support Systems** (DSS) are a form of management information system. They can be used by management to aid in the making of unstructured decisions, where it is not obvious how to work out the answer.

**Executive Information Systems** (EIS) are a type of DSS and take the form of PCs on executives' desks linked to the organization's computer network.

## 3.8 Nurse management systems or nursing information systems

Currently there are 32 nurse management systems available. As there are no central records, it has been estimated by Greenhalgh (1993) that approximately 250 sites have adopted one system or another. Few of the sites have fully implemented their systems – most have implemented either part of the system or the whole system in only a small number of wards. In practice there is no difference between nursing management and nursing information systems. Most of the systems have been designed to gather and process information with regard to workload measurement, rostering within the organization and care planning. Some provide information about patient histories and clinical records. In the UK, our systems lean towards management information rather than clinical support (Greenhalgh, 1993). Effectively, these systems are nothing more than integrated word processing, database and spreadsheet facilities. One of these systems, called Crescendo, is advertised as the UK's most exciting and innovative nursing information system. More than a score of hospitals use this system. Crescendo is made up of various modules. Each module is a program or suite of programs allowing the user to perform a particular task. Additional modules can be grafted on to existing ones as the need arises.

Managers, at whatever level, need information to fulfil their responsibilities effectively. Accurate information is central to good practice and decision making. However, good information is usually needed immediately, and gathering, analysing and interpreting data can be very time-consuming. The cost of handling, storage and manual computation of data can be surprisingly high. There are tools available for doing the job quickly, cheaply and efficiently. What is now required is for managers at all levels to be skilled and imaginative computer operators who can use these tools effectively.

With the new trust system in the health service there is a need for:

- **Senior managers** to use strategic information to plan the objectives of the organization, and assess whether the objectives are being met in practice. Such information might include overall finance, manpower and personnel.
- **Middle managers** to use tactical information, such as productivity measurements, budgetary control or variance analysis reports, cash flow forecasts and manpower levels within a particular hospital unit or department.
- **Ward managers** to use operational information to ensure that specific nursing care and associated tasks are planned and carried out properly within the practice area under their control. Such information includes number of nursing staff on duty per shift, number of patients or clients admitted or discharged, dependency level and so on.

Good, useful information is worth communicating to all nursing staff concerned but how well this information, especially management information, is received will, to a great extent, depend on the way it is presented. One of the qualities of good information is clarity. Simple management information can be cheaply and easily prepared using a word processor and a laser printer. To enhance the visual impact a colour printer and a DTP program will provide the facility for including graphs, charts, maps and so on in eye-catching colours. A computerized 'bulletin board' can be very effective in communicating information and sharing ideas.

## Suggested Assignments

AIMS: To help you identify skills for effective use of computers in nursing.
To increase your awareness of networks and associated problems.

ACTIVITY 1 You have been offered the use of a database for daily reference in your working or learning environment. What information would you choose to store in it, and why?

ACTIVITY 2 During your next working day(s) in the clinical environment, find out and describe:
(a) the type of network in existence;
(b) the practical problems associated with networks and the strategies being used to minimize their effects on patient care.

ACTIVITY 3 Read through the list that follows and rate yourself against each item using the following key:

1 I am skilled in this area.
2 I am not sure if I am adequately skilled in this area.
3 I am not skilled at all in this area.

Tick (√ ) the appropriate column

| No. | Computer skill | 1 | 2 | 3 |
|---|---|---|---|---|
| | **I can:** | | | |
| 1 | turn a computer or computer terminal on and off | | | |
| 2 | use a terminal and access menu-driven programs | | | |
| 3 | format disks | | | |
| 4 | use a word processor | | | |
| 5 | use a database package | | | |
| 6 | use a spreadsheet package | | | |
| 7 | use hospital information systems (HIS) | | | |
| 8 | use computer applications to document the nursing process | | | |
| 9 | use passwords safely | | | |
| 10 | use a computer as a decision support tool via clinical and nursing databases | | | |
| 11 | work with graphics | | | |
| 12 | use the keyboard efficiently | | | |
| 13 | save documents to disk | | | |
| 14 | retrieve documents from disk | | | |
| 15 | assume responsibility for data security and confidentiality | | | |
| 16 | use a printer to produce a hard copy report | | | |
| 17 | turn the printer on and off | | | |
| 18 | load paper into the printer | | | |
| 19 | change a ribbon, cartridge or toner in a printer if help is not available | | | |
| 20 | remove a paper jam in a printer if help is not available | | | |
| 21 | follow a procedure for the destruction of paper reports | | | |
| 22 | produce a screen dump | | | |
| 23 | initiate and maintain a manual backup system | | | |
| 24 | communicate nursing information needs to computer personnel | | | |

ACTIVITY 4 Using information given in the previous units and from your reading and personal experience, consider how the above computer skills and knowledge would help you meet the requirements of the Patients' Charter.

## Endnote

Now that you have completed this unit, you should be able to:

- explain what a word processor, spreadsheet and database are;
- outline the advantages of word processing over traditional typing using an electric typewriter;
- list the major characteristics of a database management system;
- explain what is meant by LAN and WAN, electronic mail, expert systems and nurse management systems;
- itemize the advantages and disadvantages of e-mail;
- identify personal computer knowledge and skills for the effective use of computers in nursing;
- explain how computer literacy can help health professionals to meet some of the requirements of the Patient's Charter.

# Self-Assessment Test for Unit 4

## Instructions

Answer the following questions. Decide how confident you feel about each of your answers and mark your score in the column provided or on a piece of paper. The weighting for each question is shown in the right-hand column. When you have answered all the questions, add up your marks. Then look at the scoreometer to determine your rating.

| No. | Question | Expected Score | Actual Score |
|---|---|---|---|
| 1 | List the five basic components of a computer. *(1 mark each)* | 5 | |
| 2 | Name six input devices. *(1 mark each)* | 6 | |
| 3 | (a) What is meant by output? *(1 mark)*<br>(b) Name three output devices. *(1 mark each)* | 4 | |
| 4 | Give two reasons for saving work done using a word processor on to storage media such as disks or tapes. *(1 mark each)* | 2 | |
| 5 | Explain the following types of memory *(1 mark each)*:<br>(a) RAM<br>(b) ROM<br>(c) PROM<br>(d) EPROM | 4 | |
| 6 | How can a bar code system be used in clinical areas? | 1 | |
| 7 | Occasionally a computer screen may be referred to as a CRT. What does this abbreviation stand for? | 1 | |
| 8 | What is meant by the following terms? *(1 mark each)*<br>(a) Input<br>(b) ASCII<br>(c) Byte<br>(d) Interface<br>(e) Menu | 5 | |
| | **Total score** | **28** | |

## Scoreometer

**26 to 28** You can skip this unit if you are absolutely confident with your answers.
**14 to 25** You should at least survey this unit.
**7 to 13** You would be well advised to read relevant sub-sections of this unit.
**0 to 6** You would benefit from reading the whole unit.

# UNIT 4
# How does a computer work?

A digital computer consists of five basic parts:

- input devices;
- processors;
- temporary memory;
- permanent memory (storage);
- output devices.

## GLOSSARY OF TERMS 15

**Input** is the information you provide to the computer.

An **input device** is a piece of hardware for inputting information into the computer, e.g. keyboard, mouse.

## 4.1 Input and input devices

Input is information you provide to the computer. When you type your access code for a bank's cash machine you are providing input to a very large computer system. Most input to a computer is via the keyboard (Figure 4.2), which is similar to that

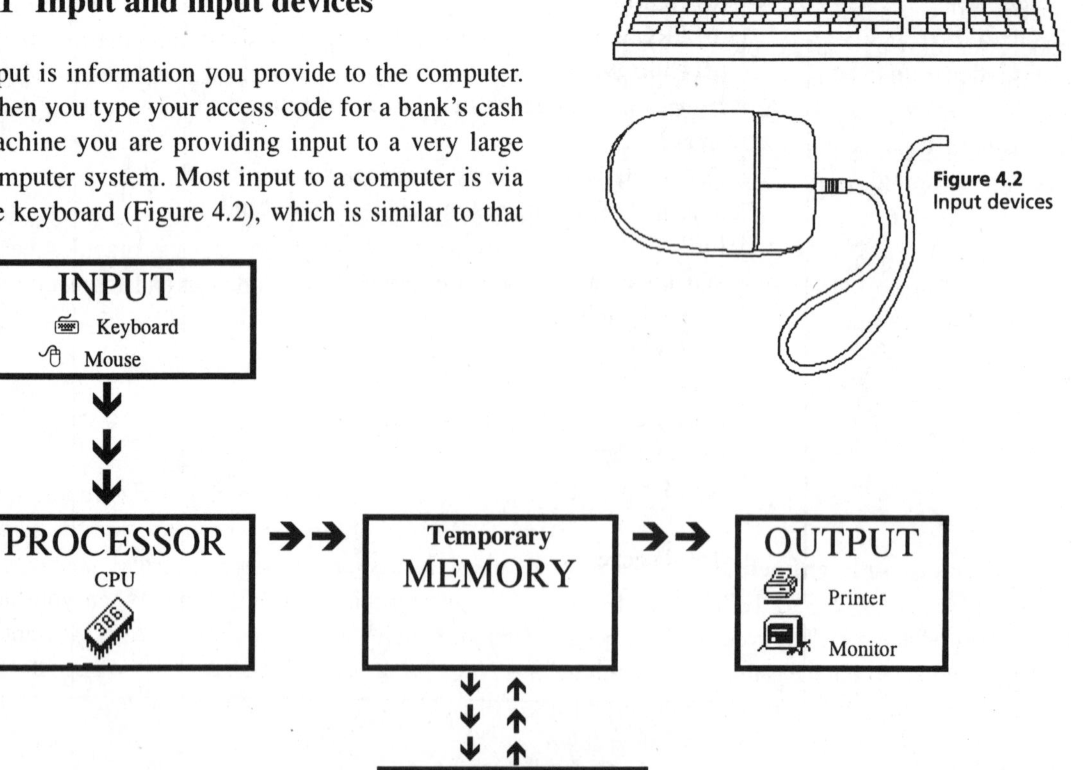


Figure 4.2 Input devices

**Figure 4.1** Organization of a simple computer with one CPU and input/output devices

found on typewriters. You do not require any formal typist training to use it. However, you will need to be able to find specific keys. The keyboard is one means by which you communicate with your computer. The information or instructions you type are displayed on the computer screen so that you can check that you have in fact input what you intended.

The computer keyboard is only one of several **input devices** or mechanisms. A second input device is called a mouse (Figure 4.2). This is made of plastic and is about the size of a pack of cards. It is usually attached to the computer by a long wire which looks like a tail: hence the name. On top of the mouse there are one or more buttons which you can press. Usually, underneath there is a ball that rolls when the mouse is moved on the desk. This action causes a pointer (often drawn as an arrow) to move in a corresponding direction on the computer screen. By pointing the arrow to objects or wording on the screen and clicking one of the buttons on the mouse you can tell the computer to carry out certain activities.

Other input devices with great potential for health care computer systems are:

- touch screens;
- light pens;
- voice activators;
- bar code readers;
- scanners.

**VDU touch screens and light pens**

VDU touch screens are generally light- or heat-sensitive. A list of items is displayed on the screen for the user to choose. A choice is made by touching the area required with a finger or with a light pen. Through a series of choices the user reaches the desired area without the need to use the keyboard or the mouse.

**Voice-activated systems**

This is a relatively new development. Currently work is being done in the area of word processing. The user talks to the computer and the letters or words appear on the screen. This is excellent for people with physical handicaps and learning difficulties.

**Bar code readers**

The bar code reader is a familiar input device in supermarkets or department stores and is slowly being introduced in health care computer systems, particularly in the area of stock control. If bar codes are placed on items such as disposable dressing packs, surgical gloves and so on, an accurate account can be kept as they are used. The ordering computer could be keeping a watchful eye on the stock level, to initiate an order for the replacement of items used when a critical low level is reached. The bar code system has been tried in the clinical area for the input of patient information at the bedside. The advantage of such a device is that the user does not need typing skills in order to input information.

**Scanners**

With handheld or flatbed scanners graphic images and characters can be captured and input into the computer.

## 4.2 Processor

When you are word processing, the computer acts as a glorified electronic typewriter, and the screen represents a sheet of paper. The text you type is arranged on this electronic page. When you have finished typing your document, you may want to print it or record it. Whichever you decide to do you will need to issue a command to indicate to the computer your intention.

Letters typed on the keyboard have to be recognized, placed on the screen and then transferred to the printer or disk. Much of this processing is performed by a chip, which is a collection of microscopic electrical circuits stamped on to a piece of silicon, made up of thousands of transistors and other electronic components. This chip is called the CPU, short for central processing unit.

The CPU is the heart and soul of the computer and is the place where all the instructions are stored and carried out. The CPU, also referred to as the microprocessor, knows what information to pass to the other bits and bobs in your computer.

The CPU carries out a certain number of processing cycles per second, typically between 8 and 66 million. One cycle per second is referred to as 1 Hertz, after the German scientist Heinrich Hertz. One million cycles per second is 1 megaHertz (MHz). So a PC designed to sit on a desk with an 80486DX CPU operating at a speed of 33 megaHertz might be referred to as a 33MHz 486DX desktop.

Besides processing words, the computer is also able to do complicated arithmetical operations at extraordinary speed. Calculations such as addition, subtraction, division, multiplication and other logical operations are carried out by the CPU.

The section of the CPU which deals with calculations is called the arithmetic-logic unit or **ALU** for short. While data are being computed they and their results are kept in special memory circuits called **registers**. The stored data and results are finally transferred to the memory unit or the output unit. Thus, registers are an important part of the CPU.

## 4.3 Temporary memory

When the computer receives an input, in order to process, memorize and store the information the computer converts it into digits, using the binary system. This is because the binary number system uses only two symbols, a '0' and a '1', to make up its numbers. This is handy because fixed DC voltages can be used to represent a 1 or a 0 (i.e. one state can represent 'on' and the other 'off').

Pictures or letters on the screen are created by points of light, known as **pixels**, that are either illuminated or not. However, what you type as input

### GLOSSARY OF TERMS 16

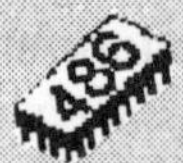


A **chip** is a collection of microscopic electrical circuits stamped on to a piece of silicon, made up of thousands of transistors and other electronic components

**Registers** are locations in the computer's memory that can be accessed much more quickly than the general RAM.

**ALU** is an abbreviation of arithmetic logic unit. This is the part of the processor where the arithmetical, logical and other operations are carried out. These include arithmetic (such as add, subtract, multiply and divide), comparison (such as 'does selling price exceed cost?') and branch operations (which change the order of program instructions) and the movement of data.

**Pixel** is the pictorial element, a 'dot' on the screen. The fewer the pixels on screen, the larger they will be. Smaller pixels produce a higher resolution image on the screen.

### *FACTS 13*

There are a number of major companies making CPU chips, including Intel, Motorola, AMD and Cyrix. The makers give these CPU chips product numbers. In 1980 IBM chose to use Intel's 8088 chip in its range of desktop PCs instead of other commonly available chips such as the Motorola 68000, Zilog Z80, used in Macintosh, Atari, Amiga and Spectrum computers. Intel next released a more powerful chip called the 80286. This was soon superseded by the 80386 and 80486, and then the Pentium. These names can be shortened and some people refer to their computer by the chip it contains: 'I am using an Elonex 386'. 80386 is sometimes shortened to i386 to indicate that it was designed by Intel.

is more complicated than yes or no, on or off. To get around this problem the computer uses a well-known code system from the United States, the **American Standard Code for Information Interchange**, or **ASCII**.

In this code system, various binary numbers stand for letters, symbols or numbers on the keyboard. With three bits, which is short for BInary digiTs, you can count from 0 to 7 (*see* Table 4.1). With eight bits you can get 256 different combinations. Eight bits are referred to as a **byte**.

| Decimal | Binary | | | |
|---|---|---|---|---|
| **1** | **8** | **4** | **2** | **1** |
| 0 | | | | 0 |
| 1 | | | | 1 |
| 2 | | | 1 | 0 |
| 3 | | | 1 | 1 |
| 4 | | 1 | 0 | 0 |
| 5 | | 1 | 0 | 1 |
| 6 | | 1 | 1 | 0 |
| 7 | | 1 | 1 | 1 |

**Table 4.1 Reading binary numbers.** Because the system has only two symbols, binary place columns increase by powers of two and binary numbers quickly turn into multidigit figures. Adding up the value of places marked by binary 1s gives the decimal equivalent. Thus, binary 111 is 4 + 2 + 1, or decimal 7.

Taking each of the 256 combinations of numbers as a code, there are enough for every letter of the alphabet, both lower and upper case, as well as the numbers 0 to 9, and most of the punctuation marks. The letters A to Z are represented by ASCII codes 65 to 90. Thus when you key in the letter 'A', the computer automatically converts it into ASCII code 65. The screen then knows which pixels to light up to show letter 'A' and the printer knows which pattern of ink dots it needs to make to create the letter 'A' when you want to print it on to paper.

The computer automatically memorizes all your inputs even when they are not on the screen. It stores the information in an internal memory unit, called **random access memory (RAM)**. As the name suggests, information stored in this memory can be accessed at random as required.

RAM is a temporary (volatile) memory. The RAM holds your input until you decide to get rid of it. However, it can only retain your data as long as it receives a steady supply of electricity. Generally speaking, all data in RAM are lost when you switch off the computer or there is a sudden interruption in the power supply, e.g. a power cut. (There are exceptions to this; for example, some laptop and notebook computers have batteries that maintain RAM.) If you are word processing your essay and have to stop to continue later, do make sure you save it to disk before you turn off the computer. The amount of data that can be held in RAM is measured in kilobytes, abbreviated as Kb, and megabytes (Mb).

## GLOSSARY OF TERMS 17

**ASCII.** The acronym for American Standard Code for Information Interchange, a widely used system for encoding letters, numerals, punctuation marks and signs as binary numbers.

**Byte.** A sequence of bits, usually eight, treated as a unit for computation or storage.

**RAM.** Short for random access memory, a form of temporary internal storage whose contents can be retrieved and altered by the user; also called read-and-write memory.

## *FACTS 14*

Some computers are designed to sit on your lap and have a flat screen: they are referred to as 'laptops'. Others are the size of a thick A4 notepad: they are referred to as 'notebooks'. Computers such as the Psion Series 3 are sometimes referred to as 'palmtops' because they are handheld computers.

## FACTS 15

There are 1024 bytes in a kilobyte and a basic PC might have 640K of RAM, capable of holding 655,360 bytes, which is approximately 145 printed pages.

In computer terms recording information on a disk is called writing to disk while playing back information is called reading from disk.

Several sizes and styles of floppy disk are available. 3.5 inch diameter disk (sometimes referred to as diskette because it is smaller than 8 inches in diameter) is cased in a more robust jacket than the 5.25 inch one and has a metal shutter to protect its surface when it is not being used.

A basic 5.25 inch floppy disk stores 360K worth of data (i.e. approximately 81 typewritten pages). Hard disks store far more data so they are often measured in millions of bytes or thousands of kilobytes known as megabytes, or meg, or simply Mb. Hard disks perform read/write operations much faster than floppy disks.

A filename usually should not be more than eight characters long with no spaces between characters. You cannot have more than one file with the same filename on a particular disk. The filename can be a mixture of letters and numbers.

## 4.4 'Permanent' memory (storage)

Let us for a moment imagine that you are using your computer to do word processing and you started typing a 2000 word report or assignment. Half way through the assignment you want to stop and continue tomorrow. To preserve what you have typed so far you will need to store your work before you switch off the computer.

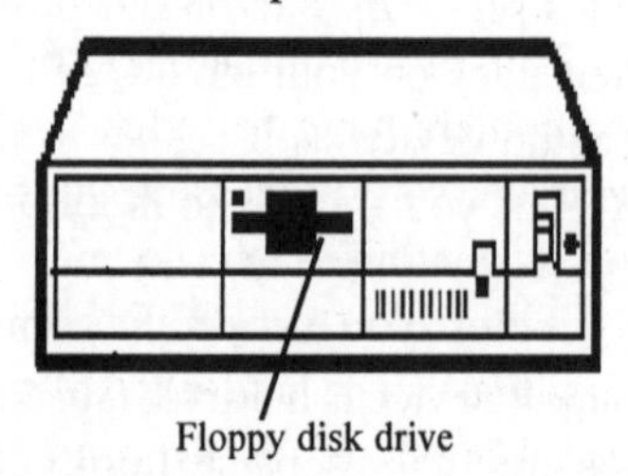


**Figure 4.3** A computer base unit

Several devices exist for storing data on a more 'permanent' basis. The best known is the floppy disk. This is a thin circular plastic disk with a magnetic coating, housed inside a rectangular jacket. The floppy disk records information (in this case your data) just like a music tape would record sound. To record your data, the formatted floppy disk is inserted into the appropriate disk drive (Figure 4.3). The floppy disk revolves at very high speed inside the disk drive and the recording head inside the disk drive moves across the surface somewhat like a record player.

In addition to floppy disks, many computers use hard disks or hard drives. These are rigid metal disks, usually fixed inside the computer. As with the RAM, the amount of data that can be held on a disk is measured in kilobytes and megabytes. Each disk drive has a letter. In a computer with two floppy disk drives and two hard disks, the first floppy drive is A and the second floppy is B, the first hard disk is C and the second is D.

Information that is stored on disk is grouped together in files. So for you to store your partially

## GLOSSARY OF TERMS 18

**ROM** is short for read only memory. It is a permanent internal memory containing data or operating instructions that can be read but not altered by the user.

**PROM** is short for programmable read only memory. It is the same as ROM except that it is programmed by the user instead of the manufacturer.

**EPROM** is short for erasable programmable read only memory. This is the same as PROM except that the information can be erased and the chip reprogrammed.

**Output** is the information the computer gives out in response to input.

An **output device** is a piece of hardware for storing or displaying information, e.g. disk drive, monitor, printer.

typed work on disk you need to issue the 'save' command. Normally this operation requires that you supply a filename for that piece of work. An appropriate filename for your report/assignment could be MYWORK1. Once the file has been written to a disk the information is retained, even if the computer is turned off. Days or even years later you can still read the file back into the computer memory (its RAM) and continue working on your report. In this case the floppy disk or hard disk is acting as a 'permanent' external memory medium to store information.

Similarly, other inputs can be stored away and retrieved into the computer RAM at a later date. Another 'permanent' or non-volatile but internal memory unit is the **ROM**, which is an abbreviation of read only memory. Vital instructions and data remain stored in this part of the memory even when the power is switched off from the computer.

As the name suggests, the information in the ROM can only be read. You are not able to alter or erase that information by ordinary means. ROM is supplied by the manufacturer already programmed. Computer users can purchase a type of ROM which they can program themselves, using special equipment. This type of ROM is called **PROM**, short for programmable read only memory. Once the user has stored information on the PROM, the contents are not normally alterable. However, information stored on an **EPROM** (erasable programmable read only memory) can be erased using ultra-violet light and reprogrammed.

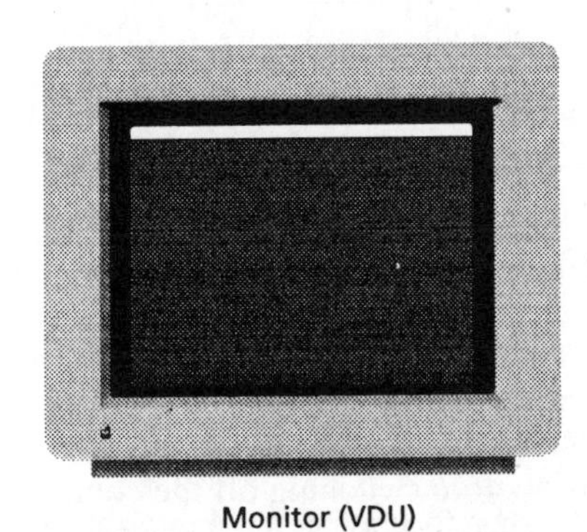

Monitor (VDU)

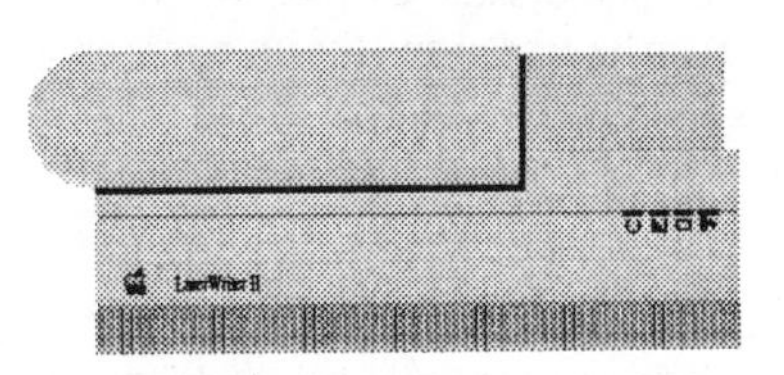

Printer

**Figure 4.4** Output devices

## GLOSSARY OF TERMS 19

**Interface** is used as both a noun and a verb. As a noun it means a two-way connection, and as a verb it means to cooperate or interconnect.

A **menu** is a list of options from which the user can make a selection.

## *FACTS 16*

Another term for the screen is MONITOR (Figure 4.4). Yet another term is VDU, an acronym for Video Display Unit. Occasionally a screen might be referred to as a CRT, short for Cathode Ray Tube, which is the electronic component that produces the picture.

## 4.5 Output and output devices

Output is the information the computer gives to you. The output may be the answer to your question or it may be a request from the computer to you to provide further or clearer input.

The computer screen is one output device which gives you feedback on your input (*see* Figure 4.4). It is an essential device as it echoes your input as you type it. Thus you are able to monitor what you are typing.

A second output device is a printer (*see* Figure 4.4). Typically the printer is a separate item, connected to the computer by wires known as **interface** cables.

The term interface is used as both a noun and as a verb. As a noun it means a two-way connection, a link between two pieces of equipment. When you have completed your report, you most probably will want it printed on paper. The printer interface cable carries the information or data from the computer to the printer. The cable can also carry information from the printer back to the computer, such as 'printer is not switched on' or 'printer is out of paper'. At the computer end the cable is plugged into a specially shaped socket called port. Most computers have several ports. As a verb the term interface means to cooperate or interconnect. For example, 'the user interfaces with the computer'. A form of user interface is a list of options on the screen from which you select the item you want. Such a list is known as the **menu**.

The menu items might be numbered, as can be seen on the monitor screen (Figure 4.4). You might need to type a number or a letter to select an item. For example to select Lotus 1-2-3 you might have been asked to type the letter L.

## Suggested Assignments

AIM — To evaluate the usefulness of bar codes as an input device in health care computer systems and recognize its limitations.

ACTIVITY 1 — Make a list of the items used by community- or hospital-based health professionals that if bar-coded would save them valuable time that could be invested in areas where computer technology has no role.

ACTIVITY 2 — One advantage of a bar code system for the input of patient information at the bedside is that nurses do not need typing skills. List other possible advantages and disadvantages of such a system. Then, if possible, discuss your list with your colleagues.

## Endnote

Now that you have completed this unit, you should be able to:

- outline the five basic parts of a computer;
- explain what is meant by input and output;
- define the terms: ASCII, byte, RAM, ROM, interface and menu;
- explain why you need to save your word processing on to disk before switching off the computer;
- evaluate the usefulness of bar codes as an input device in health-care computer systems and recognize their limitations.

# Self-Assessment Test for Unit 5

## Instructions

Answer the following questions. Decide how confident you feel about each of your answers and mark your score in the column provided or on a piece of paper. The weighting for each question is shown in the right-hand column. When you have answered all the questions, add up your marks. Then look at the scoreometer to determine your rating.

| No. | Question | Expected Score | Actual Score |
|---|---|---|---|
| 1 | What is a mainframe computer? | 2 | |
| 2 | What is the generic name of the smallest computer in common use? | 2 | |
| 3 | What is the typical internal memory capacity of a microcomputer? | 2 | |
| 4 | Which computer system is the most powerful? | 1 | |
| 5 | Laptop computers cannot be fitted with a modem because they are too small. True or false? | 1 | |
| 6 | What type of screen would you expect to find on laptops? | 2 | |
| | **Total score** | **10** | |

## Scoreometer

**9 to 10** You can skip this unit if you are absolutely confident with your answers.
**6 to 8** You should at least survey this unit.
**3 to 5** You would be well advised to read relevant sub-sections of this unit.
**0 to 2** You would benefit from reading the whole unit.

# UNIT 5
# The computer system 2

The distinctions between mainframes, minicomputers (minis) and microcomputers (micros) have increasingly become blurred because of the great advancement in technology. Nowadays, a powerful microcomputer can process information as fast as a low-range mini. Likewise, a powerful minicomputer can match up the performance of a low-range mainframe. However, since these different types of computer systems are still in existence, a brief description of each will ensue.

### *FACTS 17*

The internal memory capacity of a:

**mainframe** computer is in the region of 20 million bytes of RAM.

**minicomputer** is in the region of 6-16 million bytes of RAM.

**microcomputer** is in the region of 640,000 to 8 million bytes of RAM.

## 5.1 Mainframes

A mainframe computer is the most powerful type of computer system used for business and accounting applications. This type of system is required in order to deal with large volumes of data efficiently. Mainframes are necessarily operated by expert professionals because complex uses of commands are required for their operations.

Mainframes are used as stand-alone computer systems or to support a large network of terminals.They require an air-conditioned room or even water-cooling. The internal memory capacity of mainframes is in the region of 20 million bytes (20 Megabytes) of RAM. Many organizations do not need or use mainframes because they are expensive and too big.

## 5.2 Minicomputers

These types of computers tend to be used by medium sized organizations which do not require the power of a mainframe. Routine accounting, databases and other management information systems are examples of applications used on minicomputers. A great deal of expertise is required to operate a mini and specialist training is needed. Minis are sometimes connected to other minis in a network for data interchange or for gaining access to information in a corporate database. A mini can also function as a stand-alone system with its own database. With the growing power of PCs (see below) and with mainframes now being physically smaller than in the past, the definition of a minicomputer has become rather vague.

## 5.3 Microcomputers (PCs)

Micros are smaller than minis and much simpler to operate – the non professional can become quite proficient in their use in a short space of time. They are normally stand-alone machines operated by the end users for their own particular processing needs such as payroll, stock control, general accounting using spreadsheets and word processing.

Different models exist. Some models are manufactured by International Business Machine Corporation (the IBM PC), others are by Apple (Apple Macintosh), others still are by Amstrad and Compaq.

Micros are often linked into a network consisting of mainframes, minis and other micros for the purpose of interchanging data between operating units and accessing a corporate database; sending and receiving textual messages, drawings, and pictures; and sharing the resources of high speed printers and high capacity disk storage. The internal memory of a micro is typically 640Kbytes but this can be increased to 8 Megabytes.

Laptop portable micros are also available. They are small and light enough to be carried around. Notebook computers are even smaller than Laptops. Palmtops are smallest of all.

These portable computers might be small, but are quite powerful. They can be fitted with a modem thus enabling data to be transmitted to another computer, for example the organization's mainframe. They may be powered by rechargeable battery, but some are capable of using the mains. Some use 3.5-inch floppy disks, while others have a hard disk. They have liquid crystal or gas plasma screen.

## Suggested Assignments

AIMS To help you identify:

- prime reasons for utilizing a laptop in administrative and professional tasks.
- tasks which you do at present which could be done more efficiently by computers.
- personal skills in computer usage.

ACTIVITY 1 Laptops or Notebooks are quite powerful and handy computers to carry around. Which group(s) or grade(s) of health professionals should find them particularly useful?

ACTIVITY 2 Using information in this book and those obtained from background reading, including personal experience:

- construct a list of at least six routine administrative/professional tasks that can be done by computers.
- using the list you have constructed, reflect and identify those tasks that you personally do.
- explore if those tasks can be done more efficiently using a computer.

ACTIVITY 3 You are aware that your Department has just taken delivery of a few laptops. These have a hard disk, an internal modem, and a 486 processor. They are preloaded with a statistical program called Minitab and with Works for Windows – an integrated package containing a wordprocessor, spreadsheet and a database. You understand that these would be distributed only to staff who can make the best use of them.

- Identify existing personal skills and those you require to maximize the use of such a computer.
- Prepare a list of points you would highlight to your manager when making a case for you to be issued with one of these laptops for professional use.

## Endnote

Now that you have completed this unit, you should be able to:

- differentiate between mainframes, minis and microcomputers;
- state the typical RAM size of (a) a mainframe computer; (b) a minicomputer; (c) a microcomputer;
- outline the uses of a PC;
- identify the usefulness of portable computers or laptops in health care settings;
- identify personal strengths and weaknesses with regards to computers.

# Self-Assessment Test for Unit 6

## Instructions

Answer the following questions. Decide how confident you feel about each of your answers and mark your score in the column provided or on a piece of paper. The weighting for each question is shown in the right-hand column. When you have answered all the questions, add up your marks. Then look at the scoreometer to determine your rating.

| No. | Question | Expected Score | Actual Score |
|---|---|---|---|
| 1 | What are the obligations of data users with regard to personal data? | 3 | |
| 2 | What is meant by the following terms? *(1 mark each)*<br>(a) data user<br>(b) data subject<br>(c) computer bureau<br>(d) personal data | 4 | |
| 3 | What are the obligations of computer bureaux with regard to personal data? | 3 | |
| 4 | List the eight internationally agreed principles relating to personal data. *(1 mark each)* | 8 | |
| 5 | What is the role of the Data Protection Registrar? | 2 | |
| 6 | What are the implications of the Data Protection Act for health professionals? | 4 | |
| 7 | How can unauthorized personnel be prevented from gaining access to personal data kept in a computer? | 4 | |
| 8 | What is the aim of the Health and Safety Regulations 1992 with regard to VDUs? | 4 | |
| 9 | List the obligations of employers under the Health and Safety Regulations 1992 with regard to VDUs. | 4 | |
| 10 | List six health problems which may result from prolonged use of VDUs. *(1 mark each)* | 6 | |
| 11 | List four actions that an employee can take to minimize the risk of ill-health from the use of VDUs. *(1 mark each)* | 4 | |
| | **Total score** | **46** | |

## Scoreometer

**42 to 46** You can skip this unit if you are absolutely confident with your answers.
**23 to 41** You should at least survey this unit.
**13 to 22** You would be well advised to read relevant sub-sections of this unit.
**0 to 12** You would benefit from reading the whole unit.

# UNIT 6
# The law, data security, individual privacy and health

Although computer technology might seem to outsmart mere humans with its tremendous ability for performing tasks quickly and efficiently, it can create more problems that it solves if used incorrectly. The computer, as we know, is only a machine. While we can use it to assist us in solving problems, the results will be meaningless if they are based on faulty logic or incorrect data. In short, if we put **garbage in**, then all we can expect is **garbage out (GIGO)**.

Computers are a blessing to much of working life, but they can have adverse effects on a user's health if recommended safety precautions are ignored. The advent of computers also threatens individual privacy through the easy dissemination of information and large network systems. The computer blessing could easily become a curse, so the ensuing sections will discuss how risks to health and privacy can be minimized.

## 6.1 Individual privacy and health

With the increased trend towards centralized databanks, unauthorized individuals or agencies, popularly known as **'hackers'**, have repeatedly demonstrated how computer phone numbers, gained through national computer datalink networks, have been used to access these databanks and to obtain information that they would otherwise not have. This violation of supposedly inaccessible systems is a great source of worry when you consider the vast array of personal information that is stored in these databanks. Consider for a moment some of the agencies that might have a file containing personal or even intimate information about you. They might include:

- the Department of Social Security;
- the Department of Transport;
- the Census Office;
- the Tax Office;
- banks;
- credit card companies;
- your general practitioner;
- your previous and current employers.

Imagine what a very personal dossier could be created if all your files from each of these sources were integrated to form your individual profile. And imagine who might be able to access that information.

Fortunately, great improvements are continuously being made in systems design that help us to eliminate much of the threat of data being stolen or being read by unauthorized personnel.

It is easy, and perhaps even convenient for some of us, to focus on the negative aspects of computers and to conclude that computers will dominate our lives and turn us into numbers that are sorted, stacked and stored like objects. Some negativists believe that our society will place greater value on efficiency and standardization than on the quality of

### GLOSSARY OF TERMS 20

**GIGO** is an acronym for garbage in, garbage out.

**Hackers** are normally skilled programmers who invade systems and ferret out information on individual computer access codes through a process of trial and error.

the individual's life and argue that when humans compete with robots the humans will lose jobs and individuality.

Although pessimists have pointed out the influences and possibilities that concerned citizens should bear in mind, they do not disagree with the optimists' opinion that computer technology could increase freedom, individuality, social justice and well-being (Walker and Schwartz, 1984).

The long-term benefits of computers, the optimists would say, far outweigh any temporary difficulties and inconveniences. The time that can be saved by making appropriate use of computers can increase the standard of care and can even lead to a shorter working week for health professionals, thus increasing leisure time with no accompanying loss. To prevent the fears of the pessimists becoming a reality we, the health professionals, should use new technology with caution. This of course involves having a firm understanding of what this new technology can or can't do and being quite clear about the current legislation and regulations.

The increasing use of computers in the private and public sectors poses two threats:

- lack of individual privacy resulting from inadequate safeguards of data;
- ill-health resulting from long-term use of computers.

The Data Protection Act 1984 takes care of the first concern and the Health and Safety Regulations 1992 require employers to comply with an agreed standard.

## 6.2 Data Protection Act 1984

Whether you are a **data user** or a **data subject**, the Act concerns you. The Act also applies to **computer bureaux**.

The Act was passed to regulate the use of **automatically processed** information relating to individuals because there was a growing fear that information about individuals on computer files and processed by computer could be misused. In particular it was felt that an individual could easily be harmed by the existence of computerized data about him or her which was inaccurate or misleading and which could be transferred to unauthorized third parties at high speed and little cost. The Act does not cover the processing of **personal data** by manual methods.

Data users and computer bureaux are obliged to register:

- the personal data they hold;
- the purposes for which they use them;
- the sources from which they may get them;
- those to whom they may disclose them;
- the countries or territories outside the United Kingdom to which they may transfer them.

### GLOSSARY OF TERMS 21

**Automatically processed** in this context is taken to mean processing by use of computing equipment.

**Data** for the purpose of the Act means any information stored in a machine which can be automatically processed.

**Personal data** consists of information about a living individual, including character references, but excluding any intentions of the data user in respect of that individual. The individual must be identifiable from the data. If the data does not contain a name, but contains a code number from which the data user can identify the individual, it is personal data.

**Data users** are organizations or individuals that control the contents and use of a collection of personal data processed, or intended to be processed, automatically.

A **data subject** is an individual to whom personal data relates.

A **computer bureau** is an organization or individual that processes personal data for data users, or allows the user to process personal data on its equipment. An organization or individual may thus rank as a computer bureau (e.g. by providing back-up facilities for another data user) without actually being in business as a computer bureau as such.

Registration forces data users to be open about the data they hold. Providing they adhere to certain principles they are free to use the personal data for legitimate purposes.

The following eight principles have been internationally agreed. These principles also embody the entitlement of individuals to have access to data held about themselves. Failure to comply with these principles may, on conviction, lead to unlimited fines. Personal data must:

- be collected and processed fairly and lawfully;
- only be held for specified, lawful, registered purposes;
- only be used for registered purposes or disclosed to registered recipients;
- be adequate and relevant to the purposes for which they are held;
- be accurate and, where necessary, kept up to date;
- be held no longer than is necessary for the stated purpose;
- be made available to the data subject on request (there are some exceptions to this – for more information consult the Act);
- have appropriate security surrounding them.

The **Data Protection Registrar** is responsible for ensuring that the provisions in the Act are implemented. The Registrar has the power to enforce data users and computer bureaux to comply with the data protection principles. If need be the Registrar may remove an entry from the Register and may prosecute non-compliers. Data users and computer bureaux who feel unfairly treated may appeal against the Registrar's decisions to a Data Protection Tribunal established under the Act.

Clearly the Data Protection Act 1984 has implications for all health professionals. As data users, both they and their institution may be liable to prosecution. The need to be fully conversant with the obligations of data users and the rights of data subjects (such as patients, clients and staff) should not be neglected.

**FACTS 18**

The **Data Protection Registrar** was created under the Act and its responsibility is to implement the provisions of the Act. Its responsibilities are to: establish the register of data users and computer bureaux and make this publicly available; disseminate information on the Act; promote observance of the data protection principles; encourage the development of codes of practice to assist data users in complying with the principles; and consider complaints about contravention of the principles or the provisions of the Act.

Patients, clients or members of staff can sue a hospital and seek compensation through the courts for damage and any associated distress caused by inaccurate data or the loss, destruction or unauthorized disclosure of data about them. A patient, client or staff member has a right to see personal data of which he or she is the subject.

This section has offered some information about the Act. For further details and guidance you should contact the Data Protection Act Officer in your institution and make a point of reading the Act.

## 6.3 Data security

It is widely accepted that the most valuable aspect of a computer is the data stored on it. Given this fact, the need to keep the data secure is self-explanatory. But, as it becomes common for computers to communicate over long distances, the risks of corruption or theft of data become greater.

Keeping information safe is a big problem, largely because there is no system which is completely foolproof. Nevertheless, some strategies exist. Almost all serious application programs nowadays come with a password facility. Users are given a password which must be typed in correctly before access to the system is allowed. Individual files, or even records, can be protected and access can be controlled through passwords. For example, some users could be given a password that permits them to access files and records, write new records and update existing ones, while others could have a password that only allows them to access and read files and records without being able to make changes. Others still may be given a password that restricts their access even more.

The successful use of a password is highly dependent on users acting responsibly. Individuals should:

- keep passwords secret;
- shut down the computer or terminal when it is no longer being used;
- refrain from leaving the screen with data unattended.

Besides the use of passwords, stand-alone computer systems should be secured to a permanent fixture to prevent someone walking away with the equipment. If an application requires a floppy disk to activate it then the disk should be kept under lock and key, preferably in a fireproof cabinet. Where data is being kept on removable disks, duplicate or even triplicate copies should be made with each copy being kept in a separate fireproof place.

A regular change of passwords is another strategy which can be used to avoid any security risks – such as when employees who have had access to information leave their job. Unhappy employees may be tempted to divulge their password to others as a way of getting even. Until a better security system is developed the security of information will continue to rest heavily on data users.

Besides theft, data can be lost or corrupted in the following manners.

- **Human error.** This is the most common source of massive data loss. Data files are inadvertently deleted. By far the most sensible way to protect data from such mistakes is by making regular backup copies of all important data files.
- **Clashes between two programs.** Sometimes, one computer program may clash with another causing the computer to lock up (known as a 'crash'). Clashes occur when two programs interact in an unexpected way. If the computer crashes while in a transition state, the damage to data can be great. Just imagine what would happen if you had spent hours inputting information to your database, spreadsheet or word processor and, before you could save that data to disk, the machine crashed. The only safe thing to do to prevent a loss of data in such a circumstance is to save your work regularly.
- **Bugs.** Many programs, particularly complex ones, have bugs. A bug is an error within a program or system. Given the right (or wrong) circumstances, a tiny bug can cause spectacular data losses.
- **Trojan Horse.** Sometimes you may be running a program that while visibly performing one function may be secretly carrying out another. For example, the program could be a computer game, but while you are running it, hidden codes start destroying other programs or data files in the computer. Unlike a virus a Trojan Horse does not replicate itself or attach itself to another program, although it may be said to be a virus carrier. Two other particular classes of Trojan Horses are logic and time bombs. A logic bomb is triggered by certain events, such as certain combinations of letters being typed or the amount of disk space reaching a certain percentage. A time bomb is set

## FACTS 19

**Hacking** is a growing problem. Walker and Schwartz (1984) report that a group of Milwaukee youngsters used microcomputers to tap into the computer systems of laboratories as well as several banks and private companies. These youngsters demonstrated over and over how computer phone numbers gained through national computer datalink networks can be used to violate the security of supposedly inaccessible systems.

**Trap door.** This is not in itself a virus. It is an entry point. It may be put in by software developers to enable them to bypass access controls while working on a new piece of software. It could be used at a later date to insert a virus.

| | |
|---|---|
| **Backups** | Maintain regular backups of all files. |
| **Software** | Use software that comes from reputable sources.<br>Avoid using pirated versions of software. |
| **Vaccine** | Inoculate the computer against known viruses. |
| **Screening** | Ensure that any disk received with data is virus-free by checking it using the latest version of a virus-checking program. |
| **Compartmentalization** | Keep program files and data files in separate directories or better still on separate disks. |
| **Performance** | Any flaws in a widely used program should be investigated and rectified as soon as they come to light. |
| **Virus guard** | Install a virus guard. This will sound an alarm if any file infected with a known virus is accessed in any way. |
| **Access control** | Prevent unauthorized access to data files or programs by using access controls such as passwords. |

**Table 6.1** How to protect a computer system against viruses

off on a particular date. For example, the viruses April Fool's Day and Friday the Thirteenth were released by time bombs.

- **Virus.** This is a category of software which infects programs and data files and which replicates itself without the user knowing about it. A virus can spread via disks and the main problem is usually its side-effects. Viruses have been known to transmit themselves over an entire network. There are over 200 viruses at large and the number is steadily growing. The most serious type is the one which infects an operating system as this governs the whole running of a computer system. Fortunately there are vaccine programs that can deal with viruses. Although virus infection is just another PC problem, the more preventative measures that can be taken against viruses entering a system the better (see Table 6.1 and Facts 19).

## 6.4 Health and Safety (Display Screen Equipment) Regulations 1992

While computers are a blessing in many ways, they can also be a curse, since they can affect our health. The VDUs (visual display units) are the real culprits. They are alleged to be responsible for a wide range of health problems. However, it is important to bear in mind that in most cases the problems do not arise directly from the VDUs themselves, but from the way in which they are used. The problems can be minimized and in most cases avoided by good practice (*see* Table 6.2).

To protect those workers who habitually use VDUs for a significant part of their normal work, the Health and Safety at Work legislation requires employers to comply with a general set of objectives.

- Employers are obliged to look at the hardware, the environment and factors specific to the individuals using the equipment. Where risks are identified, the employer must take steps to reduce them.
- Employers are obliged to ensure that workstations meet minimum requirements. For example, VDUs should have adjustable brightness and contrast controls.
- On request, employers should arrange eye tests and provide spectacles if special ones are needed.
- Employers should ensure that employees can use all aspects of their workstation equipment safely and know how to make the best use of it to avoid health problems.

Employers have until the end of 1996 to upgrade

existing equipment (unless immediate action is necessary to reduce risks). Equipment used for the first time must comply immediately. See Table 6.2 for a list of the possible risks to personal health posed by computer use, and related tips for prevention and self-help.

## 6.5 Copyright

In the UK copyright is governed by the Copyright, Designs and Patents Act 1988. For the purposes of the Act, a computer program is a literary work, and copyright is infringed if it is copied or adapted without the permission of the copyright holder.

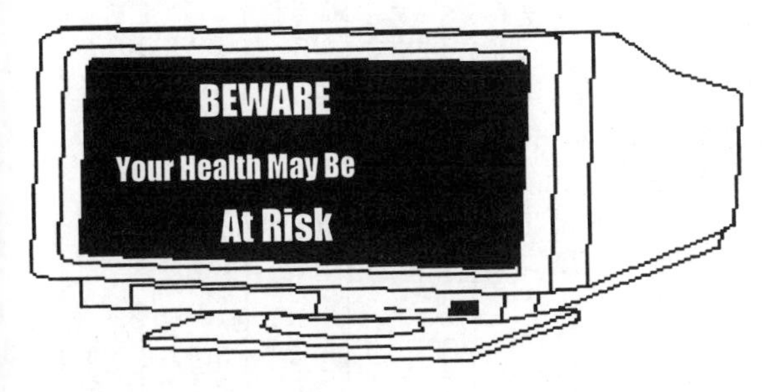


**Figure 6.1** A video display unit

You will also be committing an offence if you buy a computer program and use it on more than one computer without prior agreement. However, making a backup copy of a program you bought for security reasons is not an infringement of copyright if the software supplier gives authorization to do so. FAST, which is an acronym for Federation Against Software Theft, is an organization formed by software suppliers in the UK. FAST is prepared to bring legal action against any individual or organization breaking copyright law. If, for example, a hospital or health centre is found to be in breach of copyright it not only has to pay damages and costs, but also loses the licence to use the software. Can you imagine the chaos that would be caused in a hospital if it should suddenly lose a commercial database containing all the treatment records of all the patients?

### FACTS 20

Q. Do VDUs give out harmful levels of radiation?

A. No. VDUs give out both visible light (which enables us to see the screen) and other forms of electromagnetic radiation which can be harmful above certain levels. However, the levels emitted from VDUs are well below the safe levels set out in international recommendations. So your employer does not have to check radiation levels from your VDU, and you do not need special devices such as protective spectacles, screens or aprons when using it (Health and Safety Executive, 1992).

## 6.6 The Computer Misuse Act 1990

As stated earlier, hacking into computer systems and data is a great source of worry. In an attempt to respond to this growing concern, the Computer Misuse Act 1990 was passed. Under this Act, it is an offence if a person who knows he or she has no authority:

- attempts to gain access to a computer system (it is the attempt which is the crime, the hacker's success or failure is irrelevant);
- has gained access to another system with intent to commit another offence;
- modifies data or programs.

Note that the simple addition of data is not an offence, just its corruption or destruction.

### FACTS 21

The deliberate introduction of computer viruses into a system is an offence.

The maximum penalty for offences under the Computer Misuse Act 1990 is as follows.

| | |
|---|---|
| Unauthorized access | imprisonment for up to six months and/or a fine of up to £2000. |
| Unauthorized access with intent to commit another offence | imprisonment for up to five years and/or an unlimited fine |
| Unauthorized modification of data/ programs | imprisonment for up to five years and/or an unlimited fine. |

| | Possible problems | What can you do to help yourself |
|---|---|---|
| **Eyesight** | Working with VDUs for long periods of time can cause discomfort to the eyes, such as tired eyes and eyestrain. This is because the VDU gives your eyes more demanding tasks. | • Adjust your chair and VDU to get a good viewing. As a broad guide your eyes should be at the same height as the top of the VDU casing.<br>• Ensure the environment is properly lit.<br>• Make sure the characters on your screen are sharply focused and can be read easily. Correct flickering images on the screen immediately.<br>• Adjust brightness and contrast controls to suit the right level of comfort for your eyes.<br>• Ensure bright lights are not reflected in the screen.<br>• Adjust curtains or blinds to prevent unwanted light.<br>• Affix a filter to the screen.<br>• Take short but frequent screen breaks. |
| **Bi-focals** | Using bi-focals can be a problem since it is important that when you are using the VDU you can see the screen comfortably without having to raise or lower your head. | • Consult your doctor or optician as you may need a different type of glasses to work comfortably.<br>• Consider moving to varilux lenses. |
| **Contact lenses** | The heat generated by VDUs tends to make the atmosphere drier than in rooms without them. This can be a problem for users of contact lenses since a dry environment tends to cause them discomfort. | • Blink your eyelids more often.<br>• Use tear substitute drops.<br>• Wear glasses instead of lenses. |
| **Aches and pains** | After long periods of uninterrupted VDU use, you may experience aches and pains in your hands, wrists, arms, neck, shoulders or back. These aches and pains are usually short lived. | • Use a chair with adjustable height and back support and adjust it so that your shoulders are approximately level with the top of the VDU casing.<br>• Make sure there is enough space underneath your desk to move your legs freely.<br>• Avoid excessive pressure on the backs of your legs and knees. A footrest, particularly for smaller users, may be helpful.<br>• Do not sit in the same position for long periods. Change your posture as often as practicable.<br>• Adjust your keyboard and screen to get a good keying. A space in front of the keyboard is sometimes helpful for resting the hands and wrists while not keying.<br>• Don't bend your hands up at the wrists when keying. Try to keep a soft touch on the keys and don't overstretch your fingers.<br>• Use a document holder to avoid awkward neck movements.<br>• Take short but frequent breaks if you are going to be using the computer for a longer period of time.<br>• Stretch your fingers and body at frequent intervals.<br>• Get up and walk around. |
| **Stress** | Working with VDUs can be stressful for some people, particularly when a system is not working very well or you have had inadequate training to operate the system. | • Ensuring that you have been offered sufficient and appropriate training will help to reduce most of your stress.<br>• You should let your employer know if the system is not working well and causing you undue stress.<br>• Talk to your safety representatives. |
| **Headaches** | Glare from the screen, poor image quality, poor eyesight, poor posture, or a combination of these can cause you to have headaches. | • Use a non-glare screen.<br>• Use a high definition screen.<br>• Use spectacles if required.<br>• Use an appropriate chair. |
| **Pregnancy** | Reports of higher levels of miscarriage and birth defects among some groups of VDU workers have raised some concern. By and large scientific studies carried out to date do not show any link between miscarriages or birth defects and working with VDUs. | • If you are pregnant and anxious about working with VDUs you should contact your doctor or talk to someone who is well-informed on current authoritative scientific information. |
| **Skin disorders** | Skin rashes have been reported by a small number of people. The exact cause is not known, but it seems possible that a combination of dry air, the electrostatic charge in the room and individual susceptibility may be involved. | • Reducing the electrostatic charge in the room and increasing the humidity may help. |
| **Epileptic seizures** | Some people who suffer from photosensitive epilepsy and are susceptible to flickering lights and striped patterns may experience seizures in some circumstances. | • If you are one of these people then you should avoid working with VDUs. |

**Table 6.2** Problems associated with VDUs and possible solutions

## Suggested Assignments

AIMS — To consider the likely problems with regard to automation of data in hospital settings.
To consider the responsibility of health professionals with regard to personal data belonging to patients or clients.

ACTIVITY 1 — Imagine you are working in a fully computerized ward or outpatient clinic. Suddenly the system crashes. Consider the difficulties which could arise owing to delays caused by this non-availability of computer facilities. What strategies could be used to limit the effect of such a disaster?

ACTIVITY 2 — When passwords are issued to users a list of the passwords is usually kept on paper by the manager. The possibility of the list falling into the wrong hands cannot be overlooked. How could a system be arranged so that each operator has a password which has never been written down?

ACTIVITY 3 — Using the literature identify:

- the categories of personal data that are completely exempted from the Act and relate these to patient, client and nursing staff data kept by hospitals;
- types of personal data belonging to patients or clients that legally they may not be denied access to;
- personal data belonging to patients or clients that may be disclosed to a third party without their permission.

ACTIVITY 4 — The next time you work in an environment where computers are being used for storing demographic information about patients or clients and staff, evaluate the process used to register computerized personal data.

## Endnote

Now that you have completed this unit, you should be able to:

- explain what is meant by the terms data user, data subject, computer bureau and personal data;
- state the aim of the Data Protection Act 1984;
- list the obligations of data users and computer bureaux concerning personal data;
- outline the eight internationally agreed principles relating to personal data;
- outline the role of the Data Protection Registrar;
- outline some strategies to keep data secure and prevent inadvertent loss or corruption;
- state the purpose of the Health and Safety Regulations 1992 with regard to VDUs;
- outline employers' obligations under the Health and Safety Regulations 1992;
- describe a range of possible health problems which may result from using VDUs;
- describe the actions that employers and individual users might take to minimize the risk of ill-health resulting from VDUs.

# Self-Assessment Test for Unit 7

## Instructions

Answer the following questions. Decide how confident you feel about each of your answers and mark your score in the column provided or on a piece of paper. The weighting for each question is shown in the right-hand column. When you have answered all the questions, add up your marks. Then look at the scoreometer to determine your rating.

| No. | Question | Expected Score | Actual Score |
|---|---|---|---|
| 1 | How many characters can a filename have using MS-DOS? | 1 | |
| 2 | How many characters can a filename extension have using MS-DOS? | 1 | |
| 3 | Complete the following blanks. *(1 mark each)* The first floppy disk drive on a stand-alone system is usually referred to as __ and the second as __ | 2 | |
| 4 | What is the difference between a program file and a data file? | 4 | |
| 5 | What are UNIX and OS/2? | 2 | |
| 6 | List five types of operating system. *(1 mark each)* | 5 | |
| 7 | DIR is short for what? | 1 | |
| 8 | What would you use the following DOS programs for? *(1 mark each)*<br>(a) CHKDSK.EXE<br>(b) DISKCOPY.EXE | 2 | |
| 9 | What would you use the following DOS commands for? *(1 mark each)*<br>CD<br>DIR<br>MD<br>RD | 4 | |
| 10 | State the purpose of a directory and subdirectory. *(1 mark each)* | 2 | |
| 11 | What is the role of the operating system? | 2 | |
| | **Total score** | **26** | |

## Scoreometer

**24 to 26** You can skip this unit if you are absolutely confident with your answers.
**13 to 23** You should at least survey this unit.
**6 to 12** You would be well advised to read relevant sub-sections of this unit.
**0 to 5** You would benefit from reading the whole unit.

# UNIT 7
# MS-DOS

## 7.1 Operating systems

As pointed out in Unit 1, the operating system is a piece of software that gives the computer an environment which it can understand and in which it can function. It is a master control program which controls the functions of the computer system as a whole and the running of application programs.

An operating system performs many tasks. For example, it executes and monitors input and output operations; monitors the status of the hardware devices; receives, interprets and executes commands from the operator; implements the use of passwords; formats new disks; maintains disk directories; executes disk reading and writing operations; diagnoses disk errors; executes disk commands relating to the deletion, copying and renaming of files; reports on the status of disk usage and bytes available; and many more.

Although there are a number of operating systems, such as UNIX, OS/2 and Windows NT, in this text the focus will be on Microsoft Disk Operating System (MS-DOS), since it is used by the vast majority of computers.

The operating system is a piece of software supplied on floppy disk. On a stand-alone computer system with no hard disk installed, the disk containing the operating system will need to be inserted in the floppy drive before the computer is switched on. However, on systems with a hard disk, or on a network system, a copy of the operating system will have been stored on the hard disk. So the MS-DOS files will be automatically loaded from the hard disk when the computer is switched on.

### *FACTS 22*

There are a variety of operating systems.

**MS-DOS.** An abbreviation of Microsoft Disk Operating System. It has a large software base and is a popular system. On IBM PCs, this operating system is known as PC-DOS. (Note that Windows 3 is not an operating system: it needs MS-DOS.)

**UNIX** and **XENIX.** UNIX was initially designed for minicomputers but is now being used on more powerful microcomputers. It is widely accepted as the main multi-user system available. XENIX is a multi-user system based on UNIX.

**OS/2** is a fairly new operating system from IBM. It has multitasking abilities, i.e. processing several application programs concurrently. OS/2 can run programs written for Windows 3 or MS-DOS.

**Apple Macintosh System 7.** This is used by the Apple range of computers. It has a graphical interface and multitasking abilities.

**IBM OS/400.** This operating system runs the IBM AS/400 family of minicomputers and has powerful facilities. For example, changes made to data are automatically recorded at all times. Should there be a failure while a transaction is being processed that results in it not being completed, it is restored when the system restarts to the state it was in before the transaction.

**Windows NT.** This is a complete operating system in its own right. It offers the full graphical user interface of Windows 3 (see Unit 8) but is more powerful. Windows NT manages programs specifically written for it, for Windows 3 and for MS-DOS.

## 7.2 Booting up the computer

As the computer is switched on, it automatically goes through a process of checking that the keyboard is connected and the RAM is working properly. Then it checks for a floppy disk in the disk drive. If there is a disk, then the computer checks to see if there is a copy of DOS on the disk. If there is no floppy disk, the computer will look for a hard disk and check for a copy of DOS. DOS consists of a collection of files which contain instructions for the computer. If the correct DOS files are on the floppy or hard disk, they are read into RAM. At this point DOS takes charge of the computer. This process is known as booting up the computer.

If the required DOS files are not on the disk, the computer will report an error and will wait, i.e. you will not be able to use the computer to perform any of the tasks described in Unit 3.

## 7.3 The disk filing system

Once MS-DOS has taken charge of the computer, it will carry out any instructions listed in files known as **CONFIG.SYS** and **AUTOEXEC.BAT**. These might include scanning the system for a virus check, and/or requesting you to type your username and password. Once DOS is satisfied that the system is in good working order and that you are a bona fide user, the DOS prompt will appear on the screen with a flashing cursor. If a menu system is present on the computer you are using, it will be necessary to 'exit' to DOS in order to get to the prompt. This is often done by pressing the ESC key on the keyboard.

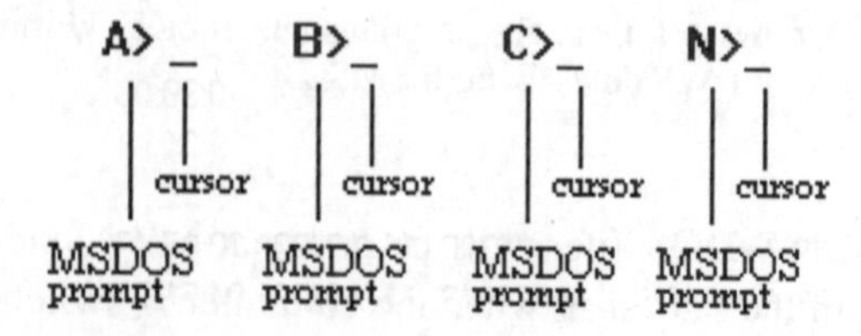


Figure 7.1 MS–DOS prompt and cursor

### GLOSSARY OF TERMS 22

**Booting up** is the process of switching on the computer and loading the operating system into the RAM.

**CONFIG.SYS** is a file that contains instructions that configure various parts of MS-DOS when the computer is switched on.

**AUTOEXEC.BAT** is a file which contains instructions that will tell MS-DOS to carry out a particular task automatically when the computer is switched on.

**The default drive and the MS-DOS prompt**

The type of DOS prompt (*see* Figure 7.1) that will appear on your computer screen will depend on the computer system you are using and the default drive for that system. The default drive is where MS-DOS searches first when you type a command. Floppy disk drives are commonly referred to as A and B. Hard disk drives on a stand-alone system are usually referred to as C and D. A hard disk drive on a network is usually referred to as N. Make sure you know how many drives there are on the system you are using and which is which.

Usually the default DOS prompts are as follows:

A> for a computer system with one floppy and no hard disk

A> or B> for a computer system with two floppies and no hard disk

C> for computer system with at least one hard disk

N> for a network system.

Before MS-DOS can load a file from disk (unless the file is on the default drive), it is necessary to tell it where the file is. For example, if you want to load a data file named EXAM.XLS from a floppy disk resting in drive A, then to tell DOS where to find this file you would first need to type the drive letter followed by a colon, i.e. A:. If the file is on drive D then you will type D:.

Note that once you have told DOS to access a drive other than the default drive, DOS will treat the last accessed drive as the default drive until the computer is rebooted or until you ask DOS to

Figure 7.2 A directory tree

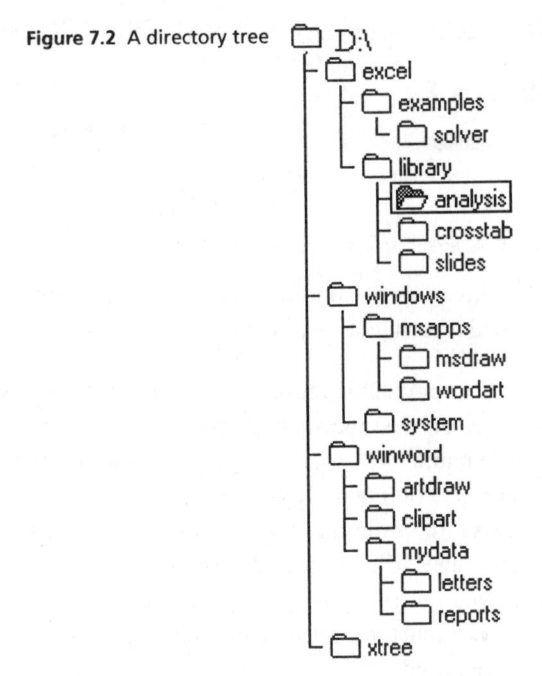


## GLOSSARY OF TERMS 23

A **filename** is a unique name assigned to a file.

A **filename extension**, as the name suggests, is additional information attached to the filename, often describing the format of a file.

A **directory** is a table of contents for a disk. It holds names of and information about the position of each file stored on the disk.

The **root directory** is the main directory on the disk. All other directories on the disk are branches from this main directory, or sub-branches.

A **subdirectory** is a branch off a directory. This directory may itself be a branch of another directory. For example, in Figure 7.2, Reports is a subdirectory of Mydata. Mydata is a subdirectory of Winword. Winword is a subdirectory of D:\.

change to another drive. Knowing which drive you are using is very important, especially when it comes to saving your work to disk.

### Directories and paths

A disk holds the name of and information about the position of each file stored on it. To keep files stored on disk in an organized manner, they are grouped together in directories. An initial or **'root'** directory is created when a disk is formatted. This root directory is denoted by the symbol '\'. From the root directory further directories, or **subdirectories**, can be created.

A directory is therefore like a table of contents for a disk. It contains the names of your files (Figure 7.3), their sizes, and the dates and times they were last filed. Put another way, a directory can be likened to a room within a large building. Each room represents a directory and the building represents the disk. Imagine that the entry hall is the only access to other rooms in the building. The entry hall is equivalent to the root directory. All disks have a root directory even if there are no other directories on the disk. Some DOS files, such as COMMAND.COM, are usually stored in the root directory, while application programs and data files are usually stored in subdirectories.

For DOS to find your data file, EXAM.XLS, you must specify a path for it to follow. For example, if your data file called EXAM.XLS was prepared using the Excel spreadsheet, it might have been stored in a subdirectory called Analysis (*see* Figure 7.2). The path to that subdirectory is: D:\EXCEL\LIBRARY\ANALYSIS.

### Filename and extension

Just as each folder in a file cabinet has a label, each file on a disk has a name. This name has two parts: a filename and an extension. The filename can be from one to eight characters in length, and the extension consists of a full stop followed by one, two or three characters. The filename and extension can be typed in uppercase or lowercase letters. MS-

| | | | |
|---|---|---|---|
| diagram4.doc | 12707 | 02/10/93 | 22:39:44 |
| draw.pcx | 35101 | 07/10/93 | 00:38:06 |
| fact1.doc | 7642 | 02/10/93 | 19:24:30 |
| intro.doc | 4629 | 05/10/93 | 23:55:02 |
| it2.doc | 93720 | 11/10/93 | 02:17:48 |
| itbuk2u3.doc | 132846 | 11/10/93 | 04:51:58 |

Figure 7.3 File names, sizes, dates and times

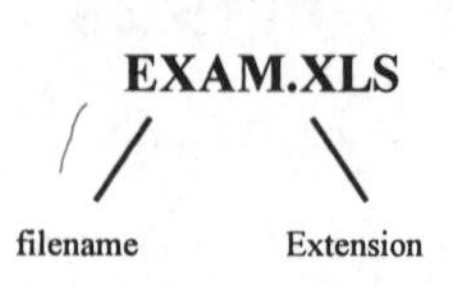


Figure 7.4 Filename and extension

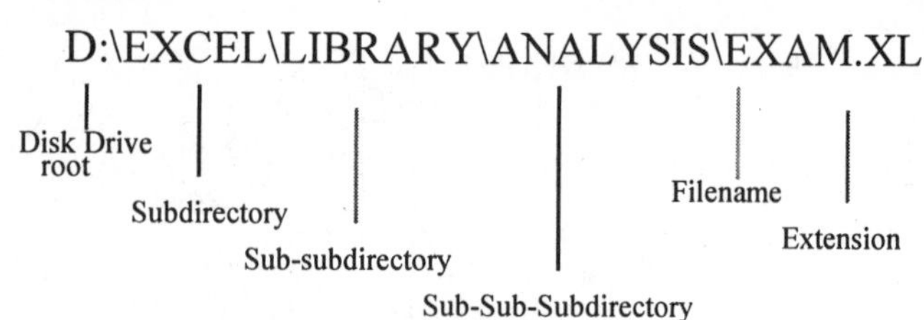


Figure 7.5 A directory and subdirectories

DOS will automatically convert filenames to uppercase. Extensions are optional, but it's a good idea to have them, since they are useful for describing the contents of a file to you and to MS-DOS. For example, if you quickly want to identify your report files, you can add the filename extension .rpt to each one. Some application packages, like EXCEL, will automatically assign an extension to your datafile. (This extension can, of course, be changed if required). See Figure 7.4 for an example.

So, if we assume that your datafile EXAM.XLS was prepared using Excel and was stored in the subdirectory Analysis on drive D (*see* Figure 7.2), the full command that you should give to DOS to find your data file is as shown in Figure 7.5.

If you do not specify a drive name when you type your filename, MS-DOS automatically searches for the file on the default disk in the default directory. There is an MS-DOS command called PATH, which is usually entered in the AUTOEXEC.BAT file (*see* Section 7.3) and which enables MS-DOS to search in directories or on drives other than the default. For example, using Figure 7.2, the command
PATH D:\;D:\EXCEL;D:\WINWORD
means look at the root directory of drive D, then in the directory Excel, then in the directory Winword.

## 7.4 Issuing MS-DOS commands

When the DOS prompt is on the screen nothing will happen until you type a command and press the ENTER or RETURN button on the keyboard. A command might tell DOS to display the contents of a directory or subdirectory, to format a disk or to load a particular application.

DOS commands must be spelt correctly; otherwise an error message such as 'Bad command or file name' will appear. You will need to retype the correct command. If you request a file that does not exist, the computer will respond with this error message: 'file not found'. And remember:

- you *must* only leave a space when it is required;
- you must *not* introduce a full stop when it is not required.

## 7.5 Running MS-DOS

When the computer is booted, DOS starts to load itself into memory. Like any program, DOS consists of one or more files. There are two files that get loaded first. If you are using MS-DOS they are called IO.SYS and MSDOS.SYS. If you are using IBM PC-DOS the files are called IBMBIO.COM and IBMDOS.COM. If you enter DIR at the DOS prompt to look at a list of files on a hard disk the chances are that you will not see these files. That is because they are hidden. This is a protection against accidental deletion.

### FACTS 23

If you want to look at the content of a subdirectory, for example, Excel (see Figure 7.2), simply type CD \EXCEL and press ENTER. Then, type DIR and press ENTER once more. The contents of the Excel subdirectory will be written on the screen.

To return to the root directory from a subdirectory. At the DOS prompt simply type CD \ and press ENTER.

After the two hidden files are loaded into RAM, a file called COMMAND.COM is loaded. This is a program file as opposed to a data file. A program file is executed or run by typing the first part of the name at the DOS prompt and pressing ENTER. COMMAND.COM is called the command processor and it handles what are referred to as DOS 'internal' commands. For example, when you enter DIR at the DOS prompt you are not running a program called DIR.COM. The DIR command is one of a group of DOS commands, including DEL, TYPE and PROMPT, that are contained within COMMAND.COM: hence the term 'internal' commands.

There are other DOS commands that are external. CHKDSK and DISKCOPY are two examples. They are program files with the extension .EXE or .COM. This means that they can be run by typing the first part of the filename at the DOS prompt. Thus, DISKCOPY.EXE can be run at the DOS prompt by typing DISKCOPY and pressing ENTER.

Data files, as the name suggests, contain data not programs. They can often only be loaded by the particular application used to produce them in the first place.

After reading this unit you should have a clearer idea of what is happening when you switch on a computer and how files are stored on disk. After you have carried out the suggested assignments below you might come to the conclusion that the DOS system is somewhat clumsy, not as user-friendly as you might have expected. Now that you know something about DOS we are ready to look at Windows™ and to see what advantages, if any, it has over DOS.

## Suggested Assignments

AIM: To acquaint you with MS-DOS commands and assist you in using some of them.

ACTIVITY 1 There are many DOS commands that are worth exploring. Some of them you should only try under guidance. Using any computer with MS-DOS try the exercises set out in Appendix 5.

ACTIVITY 2 Find two floppy disks – one should be 3.5 inch double-sided double density (DSDD) and the other should be 3.5 inch high density (HD). Now, using the MS-DOS FORMAT utility program, format the first disk at 720 Kb and the second disk at 1.4 Mb (*see* Appendix 3 for a step-by-step guide).

## Endnote

Now that you have completed this unit, you should be able to:

- explain how MS-DOS stores files on disk;
- list three or more operating systems;
- identify the root directory and subdirectories;
- state the differences between a program file and a data file;
- recognize the significance of some commonly used file name extensions;
- use the operating system internal commands to display the content of a directory or subdirectory on the screen, display the directory tree, make a directory remove a directory, clear the screen;
- format a disk using the MS-DOS FORMAT utility program.

# Self-Assessment Test for Unit 8

## Instructions

Answer the following questions. Decide how confident you feel about each of your answers and mark your score in the column provided or on a piece of paper. The weighting for each question is shown in the right-hand column. When you have answered all the questions, add up your marks. Then look at the scoreometer to determine your rating.

| No. | Question | Expected Score | Actual Score |
|---|---|---|---|
| 1 | What device controls the screen pointer in Windows? | 1 | |
| 2 | Label (a) and (b) in the diagram below. *(1 mark each)* 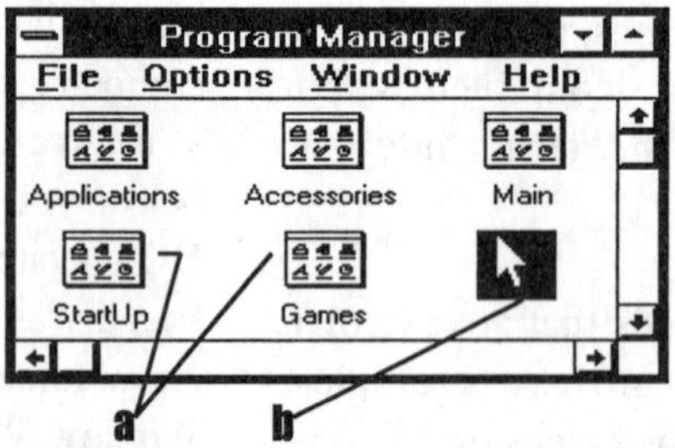 | 2 | |
| | Program Manager<br>File Options Window Help<br>Applications Accessories Main<br>StartUp Games<br>a b | | |
| 3 | What is special about the StartUp Program Group? | 2 | |
| 4 | Describe how you select an icon in Windows using the mouse. | 2 | |
| 5 | What is Windows? | 1 | |
| 6 | What is WIMP? | 4 | |
| 7 | What is the difference between 'windows' and 'Windows'? | 2 | |
| 8 | What is an icon? | 1 | |
| 9 | What is a screen pointer? | 1 | |
| 10 | What does GUI stand for? | 3 | |
| | **Total score** | **19** | |

## Scoreometer

**18 to 19** You can skip this unit if you are absolutely confident with your answers.
**10 to 17** You should at least survey this unit.
**5 to 9** You would be well advised to read relevant sub-sections of this unit.
**0 to 4** You would benefit from reading the whole unit.

# UNIT 8
# The WIMP environment

## 8.1 DOS versus WIMP

When you are using DOS the selection of files, application programs and other routines is usually done by inputting the necessary commands using the keyboard. Furthermore, the computer can be asked to do only one task at a time, i.e. you can be doing word processing or searching your database or constructing a spreadsheet. Task switching under DOS is somewhat lengthy. Here is an example of the steps you will need to follow under DOS, if while you are word processing you suddenly need to check an address in a database program:

- save word processing text;
- close down word processing package;
- load database program;
- search information required;
- close down database package;
- reload word processing package;
- retrieve word processing text file.

Each time you need to use a different application package, be it for one minute or two, you have to go through this process. Similarly, if you are using your word processor to edit one text file, you will need to save that file before you can open another text file (although more powerful word processors can have a number of files open at the same time). All this can be time-consuming and somewhat irritating.

By using a multitasking application program like Windows™, several tasks can be on the screen at the same time, avoiding the need to exit one program to access another. Using the electronic techniques known as 'windows, icons, mouse and pointers' (WIMP), the selection of files, applications and specific routines is done without the need to use the keyboard to input commands.

### GLOSSARY OF TERMS 24

**Windows** can be described as a collection of programs, or suite of software, written for personal computers and published by Microsoft. It is sometimes referred to as a GUI (graphical user interface).

**Icon** is the name given to certain graphic objects you see in the window, when Windows has been activated. They are used in conjunction with a cursor and pointer for selecting options from drop-down menus, or for running programs or tasks.

**Program Manager** manages all activities when programs are being run under the Windows environment.

## 8.2 Windows

Windows (written with a uppercase W) is a product produced by Microsoft, while windows (written with a lowercase w) refers to frame areas of the computer screen. The product Windows™ can be described as a collection of programs, written for personal computers. Windows offers computer users an 'easy' way of issuing command(s) to the computer in order to run software.

Basically, instead of typing instructions to tell the computer what you want it to do, you point to small pictures called **'icons'** (Figure 8.1) and dialogue boxes.

Windows acts as a Graphic Interface between the computer and the User. Windows itself is an

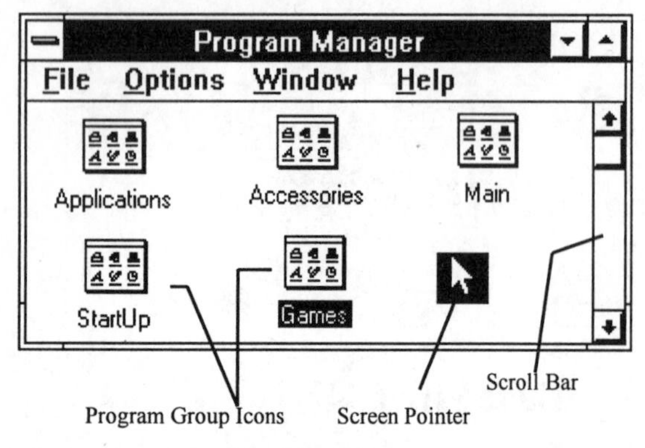


Figure 8.1 A view of the Program Manager window in Windows 3.1

> **GLOSSARY OF TERMS 25**
>
> A **program** is a set of instructions which tells the computer what to do, step by step.
>
> **Program Group** is a collection of programs and documents represented by an icon.
>
> **Application programs** are pre-written software programs which contain specific instructions to enable the computer to carry out tasks such as word processing or accounting.
>
> **Pointer** is another name for cursor. The pointer changes its shape. Sometimes it looks like an arrow, sometimes like a vertical bar and at other times like a plus sign, hourglass, etc.

application program that runs within a window – this window is called the Program Manager.

**Windows Program Manager**

The Program Manager starts every time Windows is run. As its name suggests, the Program Manager is used to manage Windows programs. When Windows is first started, you are presented with an open Program Manager window with five Program Groups within it.

Figure 8.1 shows the Program Manager window, with the five Program Groups that you could expect to see. Bear in mind that your screen might look different, depending upon the options that have been selected and the programs that have been installed.

Each Program Group is represented by an **icon**. Program Groups are like file folders, and each group contains several programs as illustrated in Table 8.1.

The StartUp Program Group is a little special. Any applications or utilities placed in this group will be started up automatically when Windows is run.

Programs can be added to or deleted from any Program Group. Program Groups can be opened and closed as required. When Program Groups are opened their contents are displayed in their relative windows, as shown in Figure 8.2. The Program Group windows can be opened, closed, moved and sized as required. A window that is too small to display all its contents – like the Applications and Accessories windows in Figure 8.2 – has scroll bars to allow you to scroll the window to view the hidden contents. The Main and Games windows in Figure 8.2 have no hidden contents, and hence no scroll bars.

Usually in a well-organized Program Manager window only one of the Program Group windows is kept opened. All the other Program Group windows are minimized and appear as Program Group icons (*see* Figure 8.3.)

| The Applications Program Group | The Accessories Program Group | The Main Program Group | The Games Program Group |
|---|---|---|---|
| Contains application programs (e.g. Word, Excel, Ami Pro) that are bought separately. | Contains Windows' own word processing, drawing, communications and multimedia programs. | Contains utilities to maintain the Windows environment and organize files. | Contains computer games. |

Table 8.1 Program Groups

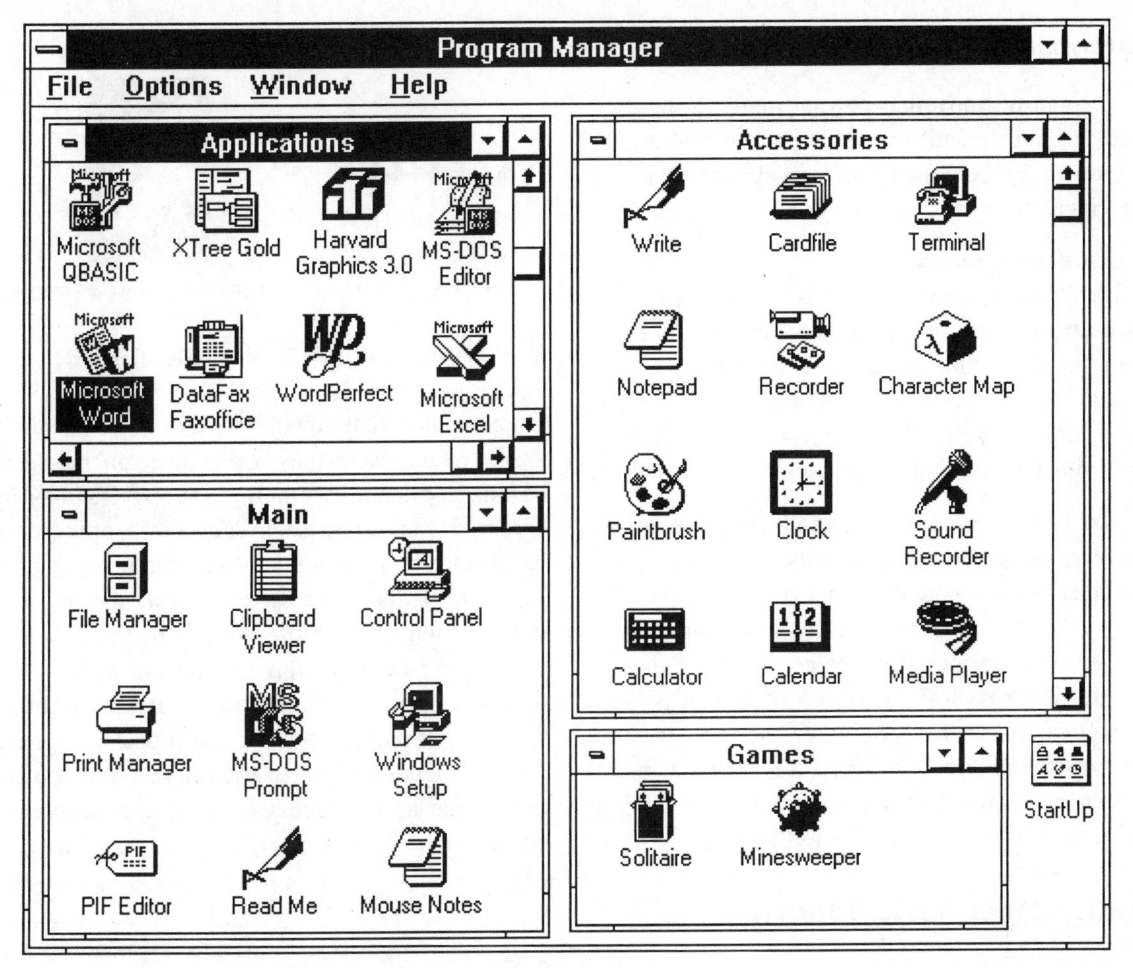


**Figure 8.2** The Program Manager with four Program Groups opened

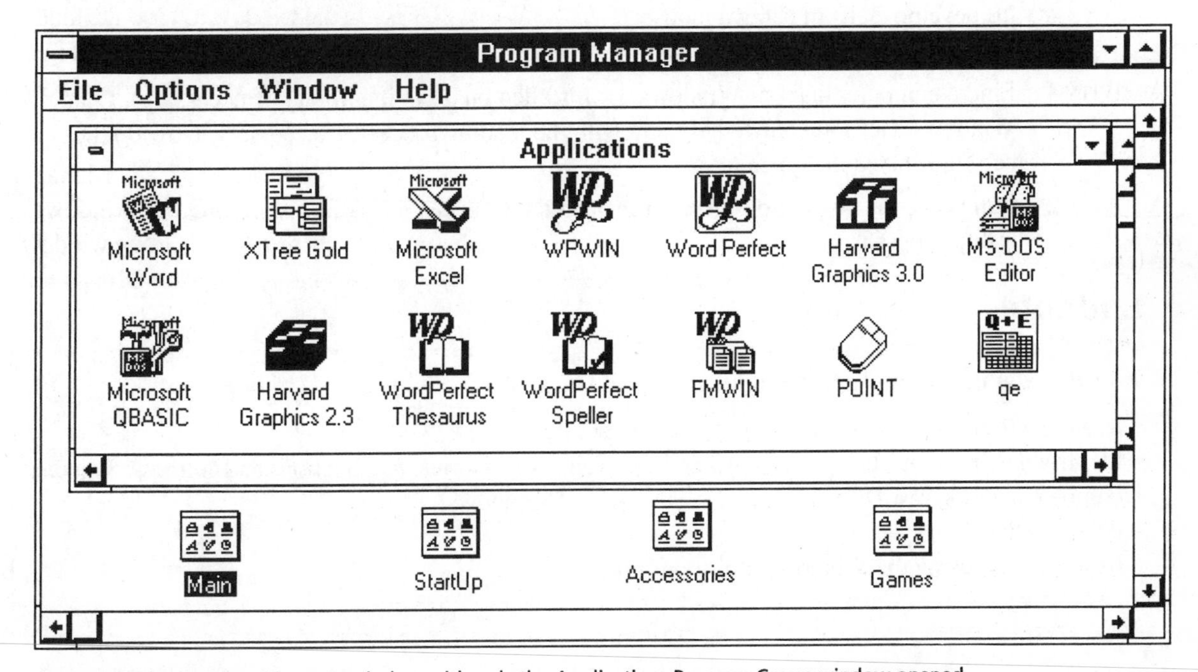


**Figure 8.3** The Program Manager window with only the Applications Program Group window opened.

Icons can be moved from one place to another. Moving icons and opening, closing and sizing windows can be done using the keyboard, but it is much easier to use a mouse.

**Input device: mouse**

With Windows some commands are much easier to issue with a mouse. The mouse has one or more buttons on it. Most mice work by rolling a ball, which is situated underneath it, across a flat surface or a 'mouse pad'. The pointer (Figure 8.5) is controlled by moving the mouse.

If you have never used a mouse before, you might have some difficulties initially. However, with practice you are bound to improve your skill. The way to use the mouse is to place your hand on top and move it across a flat surface. When the mouse is moved across a flat surface, the screen pointer moves across the computer screen in the corresponding direction. An icon is selected on the screen by pointing to it and then pressing or clicking the mouse button (usually the left button).

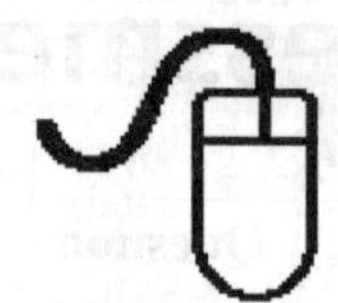

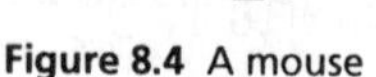

**Figure 8.4** A mouse

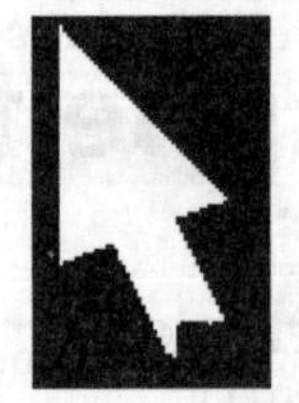

**Figure 8.5** The screen pointer

## 8.3 Menus: drop-down and pop-up

On computers that do not have Windows installed, a fixed menu system may be displayed on the screen so that applications running under DOS may be accessed with some ease. In such a case, options can be selected by pressing the suggested button on the keyboard. If the menu system allows the use of a mouse, then moving the pointer to the required option and clicking the left button selects the required option. A variation on the fixed menu system is the drop-down or pop-up menu. These types of menus are hidden and can be brought on to the screen as required by pressing a particular button on the keyboard.

## Suggested Assignments

AIMS
To acquaint you with Windows environment.
To develop skills in using a mouse.
To practice formatting disks using the Windows utility program.

ACTIVITY 1
Find a computer that has Windows 3.1 installed on it (visit a library, if necessary). Load Windows. Get someone to help you with the loading process, if necessary. Now do the activities listed in Appendix 4.

ACTIVITY 2
Following the instructions given in Appendix 3, format a disk or disks using the Windows utility program.

## Endnote

Now that you have completed this unit, you should be able to:

- identify Program Groups, icons and the screen pointer;
- identify the Program Manager window and the Main, Accessories, Applications and Games windows;
- compare and contrast DOS commands with those of Windows;
- define WIMP;
- format a disk using the Windows utility program.

# Self-Assessment Test for Unit 9

## Instructions

Answer the following questions. Decide how confident you feel about each of your answers and mark your score in the column provided or on a piece of paper. The weighting for each question is shown in the right-hand column. When you have answered all the questions, add up your marks. Then look at the scoreometer to determine your rating.

| No. | Question | Expected Score | Actual Score |
|---|---|---|---|
| 1 | What is a query language? | 2 | |
| 2 | Name seven high-level computer languages. *(1 mark each)* | 7 | |
| 3 | Explain what is meant by a low-level computer language. | 2 | |
| 4 | Name nine common errors made by users when entering commands into a computer. *(1 mark each)* | 9 | |
| 5 | What does the word BASIC stand for? | 1 | |
| 6 | What does COBOL stand for? | 1 | |
| 7 | What does FORTRAN stand for? | 1 | |
| | **Total score** | **23** | |

## Scoreometer

**21 to 23** You can skip this unit if you are absolutely confident with your answers.
**12 to 20** You should at least survey this unit.
**6 to 11** You would be well advised to read relevant sub-sections of this unit.
**0 to 5** You would benefit from reading the whole unit.

# UNIT 9
# Communicating with computers

## 9.1 Issuing commands

When you use a computer, the way you communicate with it is of vital importance. Computers need proper instructions before they can perform any task. They rigidly follow any set of instructions to the letter. The computer receives its instructions from the software and from you, the user. If the instructions are incomprehensible, then the computer is unable to respond or will respond in an erratic manner. Over 50 per cent of the frustration associated with using computers is due to user errors. It should always be borne in mind that just as we human beings have our own languages, computers too have their own languages. Just as we have our own idiosyncratic preferences, computers will only accept instructions in a particular format. So, in order to communicate effectively with these machines, it is important that you use the language that they understand. If you have entered an instruction incorrectly, no amount of frantic ill-treatment of the keyboard or abusive language is likely to intimidate the computer into responding in the manner you wish, since it cannot see your non-verbal messages or hear your verbal abuses.

Most of the communication with the computer is via the keyboard or mouse. If you type garbage, then you can expect the computer to respond with garbage. The computer is not very forgiving. For example, if you put a space or a punctuation mark where there should be none, either the computer will respond with an error message or the program will crash or 'hang'. This can be very infuriating and can create unconscious frustration and resentment. In some cases this might even colour your attitude to the computer. So, when you are typing a command for the computer to obey, you should be doubly careful. See Facts 24 for some common errors when entering commands. If you can avoid making these errors you will enjoy working with computers much more.

### *FACTS 24*

The following are some of common errors when entering commands

- Command incorrectly spelt.
- Text is in uppercase when lowercase was required.
- Text is in lowercase when uppercase was required.
- Space has been inserted between characters or words when none was required.
- No space has been left between characters or words when it was a requirement.
- The wrong keys on the keyboard have been pressed.
- A key on the keyboard has been pressed when you were instructed to wait.
- Clicking the wrong item when using the mouse.
- Clicking the wrong button on the mouse.

When a command has been entered incorrectly, in most cases the computer will make an attempt to alert you. The computer will display an error message on the screen or make a beep.

**The keyboard**

The basic keys on the computer keyboard are arranged in the familiar QWERTY style found on typewriters. However, most keys are repeatable, i.e. if you hold down a key the computer will continuously print on the screen the character corresponding to that key, until the key is released.

To avoid confusing the computer, it is important that you do not inadvertently rest your finger(s) on any keys for longer than necessary.

## 9.2 Computer languages

On most occasions we communicate with the computer via the application software we happen to be using at the time. Like any other type of software, application programs are written by programmers using one of several computer languages. Computer languages can be grouped as follows:

- machine languages;
- assembly languages;
- high-level languages;
- query languages.

### Machine languages

These are the lowest level of computer languages. They are so called because they are closest to what the machine can understand. In machine languages information is represented by a series of binary codes: zeros and ones. A '0' represents one state and a '1' represents the opposite state. By using a combination of zeros and ones in various permutations, instructions are passed to the computer. Because machine code is the computer's 'native' language, programs written using it run very quickly. Programming in machine languages is almost a thing of the past because writing a program as a series of numbers is extremely difficult and time-consuming.

### Assembly languages

These, too, are low-level languages. Instead of being written in zeros and ones, the program is written in 'mnemonics', which are short codes that give instructions to the computer. For example, the code 'ADD AL,3' adds 3 to the value in the register AL (*see* Section 4.2 for registers). These instructions are individually simple and close to machine code.

## FACTS 25

High-level languages include:

**BASIC** This is most commonly used on micro computers. It is an acronym of Beginners All-purpose Symbolic Instruction Code. Several enhanced versions of BASIC are available.

**COBOL** is most commonly used for business applications on mainframe computers. It is an acronym of COmmon Business Oriented Language.

**Pascal** is well-suited to the structured programming technique.

**FORTRAN** (FORmula TRANslator) is most commonly used for scientific applications.

**Prolog** is a programming language that is used to write programs having 'artificial intelligence'.

**C** is a language that was originally developed for the UNIX operating system. It combines high-level language capabilities with the ability to address hardware (like assembly language).

**Modula-2** is a language designed by Niklaus Wirth in the late 1970s as a successor to Pascal and Modula. It is suitable for people with little or no programming experience following a taught course.

Using a program called an **assembler**, the computer translates the assembly code into machine code. The machine code translation of the program is then saved in a new file. When the computer next runs the program it does not need to translate any of the instructions, and so execution is rapid. Assembly language is more difficult to use than a high-level language, although it usually results in faster and shorter programs.

### High-level languages

In high-level languages the codes that are used contain more complex instructions than those in assembly language. Instructions that would need many lines of code in assembly language can be written in one line, or even with only one word. For example, in BASIC the command 'WRITE' followed by a filename instructs the computer to write data to the file. This command requires a lot of machine code, so using the high-level language is much easier than using assembly or machine language. Facts 25 lists some commonly used high-level languages. Although BASIC is an old language, it is the most commonly used on microcomputers. Its popularity is due to the fact that it is easy to learn, and some modern versions are quite powerful.

Once a program is written in interpreted BASIC, every time the computer runs the program it has to translate (or interpret) each statement so that it can carry out the necessary function using routines written in the computer's internal language – machine code. This translation process necessarily slows the computer down.

However, if a program written in BASIC is passed through a compiler – which is a translator program – the compiler converts the program into machine codes. Saving and running the machine code version of the program means that the computer is able to understand the instructions instantly, with no need for conversion. Thus, the computer responds more quickly to the instructions.

**Query languages**

Using a query language the user does not need programming skills to instruct the computer to perform certain functions. Unlike the other three types of languages, query languages use English-like sentences.

An example of a query command is 'Search patients file. If operation is hysterectomy in 1992 print name.' This instruction will get the computer to list the names of all patients who have had a hysterectomy in 1992. As can be seen, the request is made in English. Query languages require more computer memory.

Whether a low- or high-level language is used to write a program depends upon the application required. Different types of language are needed for different purposes. The popularity of a language is no proof of its merit. Fashion and timing affect what languages become widely used.

Of the languages described above, query languages have definite advantages over the rest. As computer power becomes less and less expensive, the use of query languages as primary programming languages will increase.

## Suggested Assignments

AIM: To identify a framework for evaluating application and educational software.

ACTIVITY 1 You are a manager in a health centre where an in-house programmer is in post. He has just developed a computer program for monitoring staff activities. Make a list of the characteristics that must be present for you to regard the program as user friendly. If other colleagues are interested in this project then take a group approach. (For a full evaluation of an application program, turn to Appendix 7.)

ACTIVITY 2 Assume you are a teacher-practitioner. You have just received a computer-assisted learning package which your organization or department is thinking of buying. What criteria would you use to assess the suitability of this computer package? Using information obtained from your reading, and if possible enlisting the help of your colleagues, devise a checklist, then turn to Appendix 8 and compare your list with mine.

## Endnote

Now that you have completed this unit, you should be able to:

- list five or more common errors made by users when communicating with computers;
- list four or more high-level languages;
- outline the four groups of languages;
- devise a checklist for evaluating application and educational software;
- state what BASIC stands for.

# Self-Assessment Test for Unit 10

## Instructions

Answer the following questions. Decide how confident you feel about each of your answers and mark your score in the column provided or on a piece of paper. The weighting for each question is shown in the right-hand column. When you have answered all the questions, add up your marks. Then look at the scoreometer to determine your rating.

| No. | Question | Expected Score | Actual Score |
|---|---|---|---|
| 1 | List five research activities that can be faciliatated by computers. *(1 mark each)* | 5 | |
| 2 | List five databases that are useful for research in nursing. *(1 mark each)* | 5 | |
| 3 | What is meant by input errors and programming errors? *(1 mark each)* | 2 | |
| 4 | What arithmetic operation is represented by each of these symbols? *(1 mark each)*<br>(a) <<br>(b) ><br>(c) * | 3 | |
| 5 | Name two statistical packages available for computer analysis of nursing data. | 2 | |
| 6 | How can WordPerfect be used in qualitative analysis of data? | 1 | |
| 7 | A microcomputer cannot be used for data analysis because it does not have enough memory. True or false? | 1 | |
| | **Total score** | **19** | |

## Scoreometer

**18 to 19** You can skip this unit if you are absolutely confident with your answers.
**10 to 17** You should at least survey this unit.
**5 to 9** You would be well advised to read relevant sub-sections of this unit.
**0 to 4** You would benefit from reading the whole unit.

# UNIT 10
# Applying computers in nursing research

## 10.1 Computers in health care

Computers are becoming common objects in health care settings. These machines are being used to calculate laboratory results, monitor patient responses (vital signs, fluid balance, cardiac arrythmias and so on) and store data such as patient records, nursing notes and nursing care plans. Community psychiatric nurses and midwives are using computers to record their contacts with clients. GPs are using computers for financial records, billing and patient-care information. In the near future health professionals will commonly use computers to generate diagnoses (nursing or medical) and develop care plans based on these diagnoses. The data being computerized by health care systems hold many opportunities for clinical research.

## 10.2 Using a computer for research

In order to use a computer for research, it is necessary to learn about:

- the computer system (*see* Units 1 and 5);
- the process of computerizing data;
- the data analysis programs (*see* Section 3.6).

Furthermore, using a computer to conduct a specific study requires careful and advanced planning. The decision to use a computer must be made during the development of the proposal.

Learning how to operate computers may take some time and effort. You can do it if you try hard enough. The computer has the capacity to process your data in nanoseconds (billionths of a second) and picoseconds (trillionths of a second). Calculations that would take you weeks or months to perform can be performed more accurately by computers in seconds.

### *FACTS 26*

In a computer program the following symbols are used to define arithmetic operations.

| | | |
|---|---|---|
| + | addition | 2+2 (= 4) |
| – | subtraction | 4–3 (= 1) |
| * | multiplication | 5*2 (= 10) |
| / | division | 8/2 (= 4) |
| ^ | exponentiation | 2^3 (= 8) |
| < | less than | 3<2 (false) |
| > | greater than | 8>5 (true) |

Although computers do make errors, any such errors are almost always caused by human action rather than the computer itself (*see* Unit 9). The two most common errors in computer processing are:

- inputting the data inaccurately **(input errors)**;
- giving inaccurate instructions **(programming errors)**.

One of the great strengths of computers is their capability to perform functions, such as mean and standard deviation, numerous times without boredom or fatigue.

## 10.3 Research activities

A variety of research activities can be performed with the computer. They include:

- literature review;
- data input;
- storage and retrieval;
- statistical analysis;
- word processing research reports.

These activities can be performed using micro, mini or mainframe computers. Each activity will be described in turn.

**Literature review**

An alternative method to searching the literature manually is to do a computer search. Computer searches can be invaluable with the rapid expansion of published materials in nursing. A computer search can be used to generate a list of references with complete bibliographic information. The indexing system for each type of computer search is recorded in a manual that is kept by the computer search librarian. The usefulness or quality of a computer search will depend on your personal expertise and the efficiency of the computer system being used for the searches. Unfortunately, a computer search does not spontaneously generate a list of relevant sources. To conduct a useful computer search you need to be knowledgeable and persistent.

When conducting a computer search, make your request specific, and limit the topic and the years searched. If the research topic is current, it can be limited to the past five years. However, a much more extensive search will be needed for a topic studied frequently over many years. Examining indexes and abstracts briefly can help you to specify further the focus of a search by clarifying the years and topics to be covered. Limiting the language(s) of the sources and the countries where the sources are published can further focus the computer search.

A computer search can be used to generate a list of references. These reference lists appear on the computer screen and can be visually reviewed for relevance. The computer can also be instructed to print these references. There may be a cost involved in a computer literature search. So it is always wise to consult the librarian about the potential cost of the search. There are several databases pertinent to nursing. It is important to identify which databases to search to generate the references for a selected research problem. Table 10.1 lists some of the most useful databases for research in nursing. Some of these databases are supplied on CD-ROM and are quite expensive. Do not expect any one library to have all of them.

**Data input**

Having decided, during the formulation of the research project, that a computer will be used to handle the data received, you should be very clear about the following:

- the variables to be studied;
- how these variables will be measured;
- whether the measurement of the variables would produce quantitative (numerical) or qualitative (non numerical) data.

The measurement of variables such as age, weight, height and vital signs produces quantitative data that can be easily entered in the computer.

Certain types of qualitative data can be coded, i.e. transformed into numerical symbols that can be computerized. For example, the measurement of variables such as gender and race produce qualitative data that can be categorized and given numerical labels. Gender has two categories, female and male, and the male category could be identified by a 1 and the female category by a 0. The variable of race might include four categories: Caucasian, Afro-Caribbean, Asian and other. Caucasian could be represented by the numerical label 1, Afro-Caribbean by 2, Asian by 3 and other by 4.

Certain types of qualitative data do not lend themselves to computerization, because the data are not easily coded. Data that are gathered using open-ended questions, where the subjects' responses are phrases, cannot be easily coded. Observations of human behaviour in complex, unnatural settings such as hospitals or places of employment produce data that are difficult to code.

Any attempt to categorize and numerically label certain types of qualitative data can distort the meaning of the data and/or can result in the loss of valuable responses. In addition, analysis of certain types of qualitative data requires frequent interpretations by the researcher that the computer is unable to perform. However, the computer can still be used in a novel way to cope with qualitative data gathered for phenomenological, grounded theory and ethnographic research. For example, using a powerful word processor like WordPerfect™ or Word™, which have excellent sorting facilities, subjects' responses and phrases can be typed and sorted electronically and quickly for the purpose of grouping and regrouping statements.

The coding and entering of data in the computer can be facilitated by the use of well-constructed data collection tools. The demographic sheet (Figure 10.1) was adapted with permission from Stronge (1985) and used by the author in a study of the attitudes of professional nurses and midwives towards computerization in clinical settings and their expressed needs (Chellen, 1994) and in another study the questionnaire items in Figure 10.2 were developed as a technique for assessing learning environments (Chellen and Jones, 1992).

The data generated with the demographic sheet and questionnaire can be easily transformed into numerical symbols that can be computerized. Transformation can be made easier by including the numerical symbols on the demographic sheet and questionnaire, so that data can be entered directly into the computer. It is important that the value for a specific variable fits in only one category. If the categories for the age ranges overlap as in this example,

(1) 20–30
(2) 30–40
(3) 40–50
(4) 50–60
(5) 60 plus

## Demographic Data

1. What is your age range?
___ [1] 19 and under
___ [2] 20–30
___ [3] 31–40
___ [4] 41–50
___ [5] 51–60
___ [6] 61 and above
2. What sex are you?
___ [1] male
___ [0] female
3. How many years have you been practising as a trained nurse? ____
4. How many years have you been practising as a trained midwife? ____
5. How many years have you worked for this Health Authority/Trust? ____
6. Which type of ward are you working on currently?
___ [1] Psychiatric
___ [2] Medical
___ [3] Paediatric
___ [4] Maternity
___ [5] Orthopaedic
___ [6] Surgical
___ [7] Elderly
___ [8] Other (Please specify) ______
7. Which of these nursing/midwifery qualifications have you obtained to date:
___ [1] RegisteredNurse (SEN/RGN/RMN/RSCN/RMNH)
___ [2] Registered Midwife (RM/SCM)
___ [3] Diploma of Nursing (DN)
___ [4] Bachelors degree in Nursing
___ [5] Masters degree in Nursing
___ [6] Doctorate in Nursing
___ [7] Other (Please specify):______
8. What is your role or title
___ [1] Staff Nurse
___ [2] Ward Sister/Charge Nurse
___ [3] Ward Manager/Clinical Nurse Manager
___ [4] Other (Please specify):______

**Figure 10.1** Example of a sheet with demographic data

| Database | Publisher/supplier | Brief description |
|---|---|---|
| **CINAHL** (Cumulative Index to Nursing and Allied Health Literature) | SilverPlatter International, Cambridge Scientific Abstracts | This is a compact disk designed specifically to meet the information needs of nurses and allied health professionals. It is the database equivalent to the printed CINAHL. This bibliographic database was started in 1983 and is updated bi-monthly. It contains more than 130,000 records from more than 500 English-language journals, books, pamphlets, dissertations and educational software in nursing and allied health professions. Records in CINAHL are divided into several fields, including title, authors, publisher, publication year, abstract and many more. The commands used to operate the system appear at the bottom of the screen. |
| **MEDLINE** (MEDical Literature Analysis and Retrieval system on LINE) | National Library of Medicine | This database was started in 1966 and is updated monthly. It contains Index Medicus, Index to Dental Literature and International Nursing Index. Approximately 3000 journals are indexed, of which 200 are nursing journals from all over the world. Information offered includes title, authors, address of authors, publication year, language of article, comments and so on. It has a help facility and on screen instructions on how to use the database. |
| **SEDBASE** | SilverPlatter | This database contains reviews of worldwide literature on clinically relevant side-effects and the interactions of all currently used drugs. Over 40,000 drug side-effects and 4000 drug interactions are listed. SEDBASE is updated bi-annually. |
| **PSYCLIT** | SilverPlatter | This database was started in 1974 by the American Psychological Society. It contains citations to more than 3000 journals in psychology and the behavioural sciences. Topics covered are all aspects of psychology, including behavioural aspects of medicine, sociology, law, management and education. |
| **ACCESSING HEALTH PROMOTION** | Sue Potter, Database Coordinator, HEA Primary Health Care Unit, Block 10, Churchill Hospital, Headington, Oxford OX3 7LJ | This is a national database of health promotion activity in primary health care. It can be accessed by all whose work or study involves them in health promotion in the field of primary health care. It contains: (a) health promotion courses, workshops and study days; (b) innovative health promotion services and local initiatives throughout the country. This database can provide useful background information for those planning to implement a new health promotion service in a particular area. Health visitors and community nurses in health promotion are invited to register their own courses/services on the database. To register work on the database, to access information or to request registration forms, details should be sent to the database coordinator. |

| | | |
|---|---|---|
| **SOUTH EAST THAMES NURSING RESEARCH DATABASE** | SETRHA | The SETRHA database is in its early stages. It covers a wide range of settings, including: ethical issues in breast cancer screening; communicating with bereaved relatives in a large district general hospital; perceptions of a multidisciplinary team towards a nursing led service; exploring the health and illness experiences of Vietnamese women; evaluation of a syringe exchange programme; and studying the effectiveness of treatments for post traumatic stress disorder. Although this database will be integrated with other regional activities, currently it is being maintained by the regional health authority, with regular updates. A printout of the latest version can be requested. |
| **AIDSLINE** | National Library of Medicine | This is quite a new database. It covers all aspects of AIDS. More than 3000 journals are indexed. It is updated monthly. |
| **COMPACT LIBRARY:AIDS** | Macmillan | This disk contains a collection of clinical information on treatment, research and patient management for all aspects of AIDS. It includes the full text of articles from core medical journals on AIDS and many more. Included on the disk are several thousand bibliographical references to the literature from AIDLINE and MEDLINE and two new databases from the National Library of Medicine, AIDSDRUGS and AIDSTRIAL. On-screen instructions on how to search the database are available. |
| **YEAR BOOK 1990** | CMC Research Incorporation. | This database contains combined year books for 1988, 1989 and 1990. Titles include: mental health and applied psychology, emergency medicine, family practice, drug therapy, paediatrics, oncology, orthopaedics, cardiography, infectious diseases, dermatology, obstetrics and gynaecology, neurology and neurosurgery, critical care and surgery. |
| **ENGLISH NATIONAL BOARD HEALTH CARE DATABASE** | Carol Cooper,<br>Campus 2000 Local Systems Manager,<br>Health Care Database Resource and Careers Department,<br>Woodseats House,<br>764a Chesterfield Road,<br>Sheffield S8 0SE<br>E-mail: 01:YCL 090 | This is a large databank of support materials for education. It covers a wide range of information, such as: audio-visual materials, computer packages, conferences and exhibitions, courses, games, open learning materials, organizations, research and reports. Subjects relate to clinical aspects for all types of nursing, midwifery and health visiting, education, management, communication, health education and much more. Any health care professional with an education or training function can use this service free of charge. You can search in person on the database computer in Sheffield (by appointment only) or you can request for a search to be carried out on your behalf by telephone, letter, electronic mail or fax. This database is also available on-line on Campus 2000. |

**Table 10.1** Some databases for research in nursing

a respondent who is 30 could tick category 1 or 2 or both. Before you enter data into a computer it is good practice to have a ready-made written plan for data input. Figure 10.3 offers an example of such a plan, which I prepared for my research study, using my word processor. The following must have already been determined: the number of columns per line, and what column(s) will represent what variables and other information. Once the data has been entered into the computer, a thorough check for input errors must be carried out. This is essential in order to produce reliable findings.

Selecting the right computer and statistical package is another important consideration at the onset. Enlisting the help of a nurse-researcher who has experience with using computers and who is knowledgeable about statistical packages could help you avoid problems at a later stage of your research.

**Data storage and retrieval**

How much data can be stored in a computer depends on the size of the hard disk. However, data can also be stored on floppy disk. Indeed, personal data should be stored on floppy disks, especially if you are using a mainframe computer. It is not uncommon for floppy disks to get corrupted. You should take good care of your disks (*see* Section 2.5) and always keep backup copies.

**Statistical analysis**

Using the computer to conduct statistical analyses on data can greatly increase the accuracy of data analysis and decrease the time required to complete the analysis. However, not every research project requires a computer for data analysis. If you are conducting relatively simple analyses on a small amount of data, a pocket calculator may well be the best tool for conducting the analyses.

A number of statistical packages are available for analysing data. Abstat, SPSS and Minitab are examples of such programs. Abstat contains a variety of parametric and nonparametric statistical tests and will run on a personal computer. SPSS (Statistical Package for the Social Sciences) is available for use on mainframes and is the most frequently used statistical package. SPSS can be used to conduct numerous parametric and nonparametric analyses and to generate a multitude of tables, charts and graphs. Minitab is a very easy statistical package for health professionals to use. A good range of tests are available. It can also produce charts and graphs.

### FACTS 27

Some features of Minitab

- **Basic statistics**, e.g. descriptive statistics, confidence interval, one sample z-test, t-test for one sample, two sample t-test, correlation.
- **Regression**, e.g. simple, polynomial, multiple, stepwise.
- **Analysis of variance**, e.g. one-way, two-way, anova, ancova.
- **Multivariate analysis**, e.g. principal component analysis.
- **Nonparametrics**, e.g. Wilcoxon rank test, Mann-Whitney-Wilcoxon rank sum test, Kruskal-Wallis test, Friedman and Walsh tests.

Minitab is composed of several interlinked modules which allow you to enter data, manipulate it, analyse the final version of the data and graphically display your results. An Outfile command allows you to make a record of all the operations you perform while using Minitab. Once the command has been issued, details of any manipulations of the data, any analyses you might perform and any graphic displays you might plot are stored on disk in a text file which you can inspect with a word processor. When you come to do your write-up, information in your Outfile will prove to be quite useful.

The Minitab package contains a spreadsheet (*see* Section 3.4). The spreadsheet, referred to as the worksheet, allows you to inspect the results of any manipulations you might perform on data. To

## Assessing Learning Environments

**CATEGORY 1 – Social Climate**

*Tick one box in each of the following seven-point scale*

1.1

Staff in this practice area are:

| | 1 | 2 | 3 | 4 | 5 | 6 | 7 | |
|---|---|---|---|---|---|---|---|---|
| friendly | | | | | | | | hostile |
| sensitive | | | | | | | | indifferent |
| callous | | | | | | | | compassionate |
| unfeeling | | | | | | | | empathetic |
| reassuring | | | | | | | | discouraging |
| approachable | | | | | | | | distant |
| unhelpful | | | | | | | | helpful |

*Tick one box in each of the following seven-point scale*

1.2

Staff in this practice area are:

| | 1 | 2 | 3 | 4 | 5 | 6 | 7 | |
|---|---|---|---|---|---|---|---|---|
| facilitative | | | | | | | | obstructive |
| disagreeable | | | | | | | | agreeable |
| tolerant | | | | | | | | intolerant |
| insecure | | | | | | | | confident |
| caring | | | | | | | | indifferent |
| unavailable | | | | | | | | available |
| attentive | | | | | | | | inattentive |

**Figure 10.2** Example of two scales in a questionnaire

## Name of Datafile: ATTques

| *Column* | *Description of variables* | *Question number* |
|---|---|---|
| 1 | Respondent ID number | |
| | | |
| | DEMOGRAPHIC DATA | |
| 2 | Age group | 1 |
| 3 | Sex | 2 |
| 4 | Years practice as a nurse | 3 |
| 5 | Years practice as a midwife | 4 |
| 6 | Blank space | |
| 7 | Years work for health authority/trust | 5 |
| 8 | Speciality | 6 |
| 9 | Highest qualifications | 7 |
| 10 | Grade | 8 |

**Figure 10.3** Written plan for entering data

inspect data you simply press the ESC key on the keyboard. The ESC key allows you to switch between the spreadsheet and the command mode. Minitab will run on a stand-alone system. You need to have at least 3 megabytes of free space before installing it on your hard disk.

It is well worth pointing out again that although computers do calculations very quickly, they are not intelligent. If you instruct them to do the wrong thing, they will try to do it. Again, since computers will try to perform your mistakes very quickly, errors that you make when instructing the computer could have catastrophic consequences for your data files. When things are not going right it is easy to blame and curse the computer. In most cases, the errors will be yours rather than the computer's; so check, check and check again that the syntax of the command you have given the computer is correct. Try to work out the mistakes before seeking assistance. Read the messages on the screen, which very often will give you some clue as to the source of your error.

**Word processing qualitative data and writing the research report**

WordPerfect™ and Word™ are two of the most popular word processing packages around. They both contain all the facilities that most people are likely to need. They are available for PCs working under DOS or Windows. Word for Windows can be tuned to recognize WordPerfect keystrokes. Four of the several useful facilities are Sort, Search, Import and Export. As previously stated, using a powerful word processing package, such as WordPerfect or Word, can help with the sorting and grouping of data for qualitative analyses as well as with the preparation of data for its entry into a statistical package.

In a recent study (Chellen and Jones, 1992), we used WordPerfect 5.1 as a research tool for content analysis of written words obtained from an open-ended questionnaire. Each questionnaire was read and a one-line statement of each point made by each respondent for each questionnaire was entered into the computer. Each text line was assigned a respondent code, a question number code, a questionnaire format code and a category code. Each statement was taken to represent an item. So each one was given a code to enable the frequency of individual items to be determined. Using the powerful Sort facility of WordPerfect, all statements were sorted by the computer according to item code. All coded statements were then converted into propositions. Using the Search facility of WordPerfect, a set of propositions was then searched for emergent unifying themes. Using the Sort facility again, the coded propositions were organized under the headings of the appropriate themes. The themes were then grouped under broad headings and regrouped under subheadings.

All these steps could, of course, have been done manually, working through each page of each questionnaire using a 'cut' and 'paste' technique. Can you imagine how much harder the task would have been and how much longer it would have taken to complete? It is worth noting that we could also have used a spreadsheet program, like Excel™.

Of course, the word processor can be used to develop the research report and articles for publications (*see* Section 3.1 for additional information).

Finally, using e-mail it is possible for a nurse-researcher to send data to and receive data from researchers around the world in seconds or minutes. With such a capability, the computer is a valuable, flexible source for communicating research findings (*see* Section 3.5 for additional information).

## Suggested Assignments

AIMS: To reflect on the knowledge and skills required when attempting to use a computer for data analysis.
To develop essential skills required for the utilization of a computer for data analysis.

ACTIVITY 1 Although computers have the capacity to process research data in nanoseconds or picoseconds a nurse needs to be sufficiently literate about computers before attempting to use this option. As a health professional, you are planning to undertake a piece of research as part fulfilment of a nursing degree course. Consider and make a list of some of the knowledge and skills you think you need when contemplating the use of a computer for analysing your data and processing your research report. After you have completed the exercise turn to Appendix 2.

ACTIVITY 2 As a community sister, community psychiatric nurse or health visitor, you are thinking of carrying out a survey on 'the prevalence of smoking amongst health workers'. Construct a demographic questionnaire for collecting the following data: age, sex, brand of cigarettes, number of cigarettes smoked per day. (**Note**: a good questionnaire for computer analysis should facilitate the coding and entering of data into the computer.)

ACTIVITY 3 Find an IBM or IBM compatible computer that has a DOS version of Minitab installed on it. Complete the exercises listed in appendix 6.

## Endnote

Now that you have completed this unit, you should be able to:

- state what is meant by input and programming errors;
- discuss the research activities that can be facilitated by computers;
- outline the databases pertinent to nursing;
- construct a data collection tool that will facilitate the coding and entering of data into the computer for analysis;
- prepare a written plan for data input to the computer;
- activate and quit Minitab;
- enter data in a Minitab worksheet, save data to disk, retrieve data from disk, request the Minitab help facility;
- list two statistical packages currently available for the analysis of data.

# Self-Assessment Test for Unit 11

## Instructions

Answer the following questions. Decide how confident you feel about each of your answers and mark your score in the column provided or on a piece of paper. The weighting for each question is shown in the right-hand column. When you have answered all the questions, add up your marks. Then look at the scoreometer to determine your rating.

| No. | Question | Expected Score | Actual Score |
|---|---|---|---|
| 1 | What is the name of this object?  | 1 | |
| 2 | Outline six limitations of computers. *(2 marks each)* | 12 | |
| 3 | Give two ways of minimizing the risk of losing nursing data from the computer in the event of electrical failure. *(1 mark each)* | 2 | |
| 4 | What is the name given to the semiconducting element from which computer chips are made? | 1 | |
| 5 | List the areas of nursing where computers cannot outsmart humans. | 5 | |
| | **Total score** | **21** | |

## Scoreometer

**19 to 21** You can skip this unit if you are absolutely confident with your answers.
**11 to 18** You should at least survey this unit.
**6 to 10** You would be well advised to read relevant sub-sections of this unit.
**0 to 5** You would benefit from reading the whole unit.

# UNIT 11
# Limitations of computers

The advancement in **silicon** chip technology has moved so fast that we now regard as common what was not so long ago complete science fiction. All sorts of machines are popping up every day. All of them designed to give us human beings a helping hand. One type of machine that is rapidly becoming a part of our everyday life is the micro computer. The power of the micro is so great that some people see them as a threat. It is true that in some areas computers can outsmart humans. They are beginning to talk to us and answer us back. May be one day they will even be able to think and have a mind of their own. Until that day comes, not being able to think laterally and in abstract terms, as we can, is probably the greatest limitation of computers. Because of this inability to make the slightest inference, computers depend entirely on us to provide them with specific instructions. The programs that are written to give a series of instructions to computers must be almost flawless in order for the machine to operate. As long as man writes the programs for computers to follow we have nothing to fear. We have the machine under our control.

**GLOSSARY OF TERMS 26**

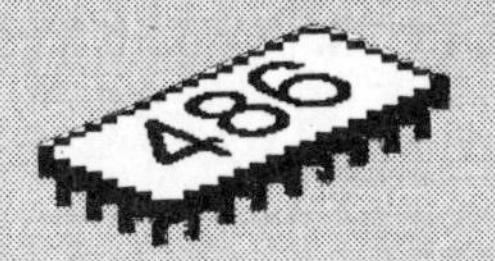


**Silicon** is an abundant semiconducting element from which computer chips are made.

Other examples of limitations are:

- electrical failure;
- mechanical failure;
- incompatibility of hardware, operating systems and application programs;
- lack of skills;
- poor quality of programs.

## 11.1 Electrical failure

Computers need a constant flow of electricity in order to continue to function. Any momentary interruption of power will cause the computer to crash. In such circumstances, data that has not been saved before the crash occurred, is lost. This can be a bit of a nuisance. Loss of data due to power failure can frustrate even the most patient person. One way of reducing the probability of losing data is to save inputs frequently and to keep and update backup files. It is, however, worth mentioning that battery backup facility is gradually becoming an integrated part of some computer systems. In the event of a sudden power cut the battery backup system will take over and will keep the computer going, thus preventing loss of data.

## 11.2 Mechanical failure

Computers do also break down for reasons other than power cuts or failures. This is quite a serious limitation, for the time lost to repair the machine and the cost of repair can be very high. The lack of access to data stored in the computer while the system is down, could be a problem, especially if there is a long delay before the system is restored. However, a well cared-for system requires very little repair. With availability of good technical support, most problems are usually solved in a short space of time.

## 11.3 Incompatibility of hardware, operating systems and application programs

Computer systems come in various sizes, shapes and designs. Although the hardware for the vast majority of computers is virtually the same, application programs must be compatible with the operating system of the computer on which they are to run; otherwise they will not work properly, if at all. The availability of a variety of operating systems (*see* Table 7.1) creates an unnecessary problem with regards to importing and exporting of data between computers. This incompatibility can even sometimes extend to computers using the same operating system. This is nearly always due to the variation in internal design of hardware, particularly the manner in which disks are formatted and the VDU is controlled.

## 11.4 Lack of skills

Increasingly a variety of input devices have been entering the market (*see* Section 4.1). Special skills are required in order to use them effectively. Learning how to use most of the input devices takes time and effort. If the motivation is there, the problem of time can usually be overcome. By and large only a reasonable level of competence is needed to use most of the input devices. For example, it is not absolutely necessary to have a fast typing speed in order to use the keyboard effectively. Although the keyboard is by far the most common input device, few nursing students and health professionals have keyboard skills. Inputting of information in the computer becomes tedious, and unnecessary mistakes are made (*see* Table 9.1). This then creates a barrier.

## 11.5 Poor quality of programs

Computers are very rigid and tend not to be very forgiving. For example, they will not accept a space, or punctuation mark when none is required. Or they will not accept a lowercase character when an uppercase character is required and vice versa. This can be very infuriating and very discouraging for beginners, especially if the program crashes as a result of an incorrect entry or the user is presented with unhelpful messages like 'error 29' or 'don't be silly'.

It is a fact that computers operate in a logical manner with no capability of intuitive leaps. They have no knowledge of the outside world (Koch and Rankin, 1987). They have a language of their own (*see* Section 9.2), with limited capacity to understand human language. All these make them 'uncooperative' and rather unfriendly.

However, it can be argued that a computer is as good as the programmer. Use of error-trapping routines can prevent programs from crashing as a result of input errors. Clever programming can build on the basic and limited capacity of computers, thus increasing their ability to interpret meanings and bring them closer to meeting users' needs.

## Suggested Assignments

AIM: To assist you make appropriate use of the computer as a tool to provide better nursing or medical care.

ACTIVITY 1 Make a list of all the routine activities that you have to do as a health professional. Now, take another piece of paper and divide it into two columns. Using information given in the preceeding units and those you have obtained from your reading, list on the lefthand column, the activities which if automated will be beneficial to you. On the righthand column list the activities that only humans like you can do. Now discuss your list with a computer literate colleague to see if there are any shared responses.

## Endnote

Now that you have completed this unit, you should be able to:

- identify a silicon chip;
- outline five or more limitations of computers;
- discuss how these limitations can be managed;
- identify activities that can be computerised and those that cannot.

# APPENDIX 1
# Keyboard layout and functions

The keyboard is one means of communicating with the computer. A typical computer keyboard is laid out using the standard typewriter pattern known as QWERTY. However, the actual positioning of certain special keys and the characters that share certain keys may differ between keyboards.

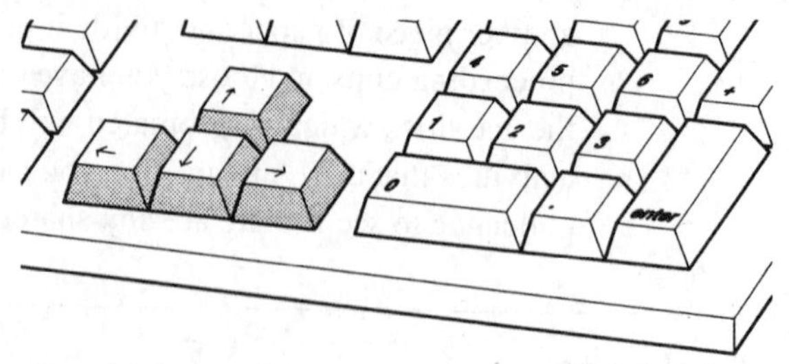


Figure A1.1 Arrow keys

A basic keyboard includes the following:

- **Ordinary typing keys.** These are used to enter data or text and may also be used to denote instructions or commands if used with special keys, such as CTRL or ALT.
- **Numeric keypad.** These are used like a calculator to enter lots of numbers. They may also function as cursor control keys, home, end, page up and page down to move quickly through a document, and so on, depending on whether the number lock key is on or off.
- **Cursor control keys.** These are four arrows (*see* figure A1.1). These are used to move the cursor on the screen in the following directions:
  ➡ right
  ➡ left
  ⬆ up
  ⬇ down
  HOME usually start of line
  END usually end of line
  PAGE UP up one screen, page or form
  PAGE DOWN down one screen, page or form.
- **Function keys.** These are used with certain software. The keys are numbered and preset to perform certain functions.
- **Return** or **Enter** key. When you have entered a command (in most cases) you must press this key to let the machine know; otherwise it will not execute your request.
- **Escape** key **(ESC).** This key can be used when, for example, you wish to stop using a procedure.
- **Control** key **(CTRL).** This alters the meaning of some keys.
- **Alternate** key **(ALT).** Like the CTRL key, this also alters the meaning of some keys.
- **Shift** key (⇧). Holding this key down while pressing an alphabetic key will give you the uppercase letter. This method is also used to select the symbol written on the top half of a key.
- **Capitals** key **(CAPS LOCK).** This is a toggle key. When it is on, the alphabetic keys produce capitals. The other keys are not affected.

# APPENDIX 2
# Knowledge and skills required for computerized data analysis and producing written reports

The knowledge and skills needed to use a computer for statistical analysis of data and for producing the final report will depend on:

- the computer hardware and accessories
- the type of applications being used for the analysis of data
- the type of research data being analysed
- the quality of the output required.

By and large, the knowledge and skills listed in Table A2.1 below could reduce a lot of tension and make using the computer more enjoyable, especially if there is no one readily available to rescue you.

| | Knowledge | Skills |
|---|---|---|
| **The computer and accessories** | • How to switch on/off the computer/computer terminal<br>• How to switch on/off the printer<br>• How to change directory<br>• How to change drives | • Use the keyboard and in some cases the mouse to enter data<br>• Activate the printer to obtain a hard copy of the results or report<br>• Load paper in the printer<br>• Change printer ribbon<br>• Format a disk<br>• Remove paper jam from printer |
| **The statistical and wordprocessing packages** | • How to input the data in worksheet for analysis<br>• How to code data in a wordprocessor for searching and sorting items<br>• How to issue various commands in the statistical package to manipulate the data such as: copy a column into another<br>• How to instruct the computer to carry out the statistical tests you want<br>• How to obtain help, on-line, manual, expert<br>• How to obtain a screen dump | • Log on to the statiscal program being used<br>• Construct an appropriate instrument for collecting data for computer analysis<br>• Construct a plan/codebook for inputting your data<br>• Check data entry for accuracy<br>• Save data to disk<br>• Retrieve datafile from disk<br>• Log off the application program being used<br>• Operate the sort facility on a wordprocessor when handling qualitative data<br>• Use the search facility<br>• Import and export data between applications<br>• Use a wordprocessor for typing the report<br>• Interpret error messages |

**Table A2.1** Knowledge and skills needed for analysis of data using a computer

# APPENDIX 3
# Steps in formatting a disk

A floppy or hard disk must be prepared (formatted) before information can be recorded on to it. A formatting program is used for this purpose. If you are using a system with a hard disk, the formatting program is usually on it. Otherwise you will need to load it into the computer. Before you start formatting a disk it is important to bear the following points in mind.

- Not all types of floppy disks are compatible with all types of floppy disk drives.
- In general, a disk must be formatted at a capacity less than or equal to the capacity of the drive in order for the disk and drive to be compatible. For example, if you have a high density 3.5 inch disk drive designed to work with 1.44 Mb floppy disks, you can use floppy disks formatted as 720 Kb. However, if you have a 720 Kb drive, you usually cannot use disks formatted to 1.44 Mb.
- A disk formatted for use with Microsoft Disk Operating System (MS-DOS) will not usually work with another operating system and vice versa.
- Once a new disk has been formatted it does not usually require formatting again.
- If a used disk containing data files is reformatted, all the information stored on it will be unavailable, although if you have mistakenly reformatted the disk, it may be possible to recover the lost information.

## Formatting a disk using the MS-DOS utility program

AIM

To format 3.5 inch and/or 5.25 inch floppy disks using the MS-DOS safe format procedure on a computer with a hard disk.

EQUIPMENT REQUIRED

An IBM or IBM compatible computer with a hard disk and one or two high density floppy disk drives.
Floppy disk(s) to be formatted.

PROCEDURE

- Select the appropriate command from Table A3.1.
- At the C:> prompt, type the command indicated in Table A3.1 then press the ENTER key.
- When requested, insert the disk to be formatted fully into the appropriate drive with the label facing upwards and towards you.
- Now press the ENTER key to tell the computer to start the formatting process.
- When the formatting process is completed MSDOS will prompt you to give the disk a volume label. Type the name you want to call the disk, e.g. Myworkdisk, then press ENTER.
- Unless you want to format another disk press N to quit.

| | 3.5" AND 5.25" HIGH DENSITY DRIVE A | 3.5" AND 5.25" HIGH DENSITY DRIVE B |
|---|---|---|
| To format: | Command | Command |
| 3.5" disk at 1.44Mb type: ☞ | FORMAT A: | FORMAT B: |
| 3.5" disk at 720K type: ☞ | FORMAT A:/F:720 | FORMAT B:/F:720 |
| 5.25" disk at 1.2Mb type: ☞ | FORMAT A: | FORMAT B: |
| 5.25" disk at 360K type: ☞ | FORMAT A:/F:360 | FORMAT B:/F:360 |

**Table A3.1** MS-DOS formatting commands

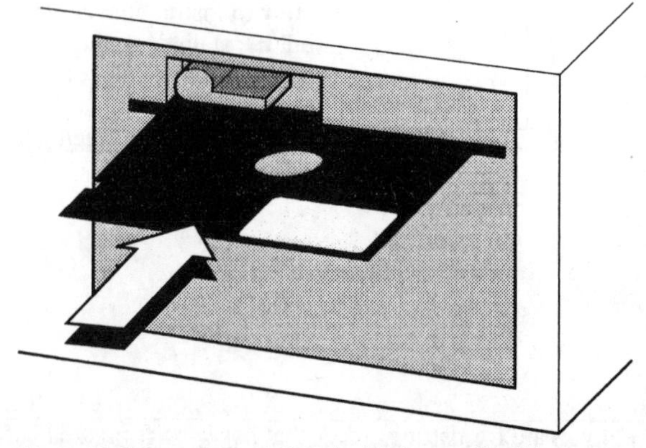

**Figure A3.1** Inserting a 5.25 inch disk into a disk drive

## Formatting a disk using the Windows utility program

AIM

To format 3.5 inch and/or 5.25 inch floppy disks using the Windows safe format procedure on a computer with a hard disk.

EQUIPMENT REQUIRED

- An IBM or IBM compatible computer with a hard disk and one or two high density drives.
- Floppy disk(s) to be formatted.

PROCEDURE

- Run Windows.
- When the Windows Program Manager appears, insert your disk to be formatted into the appropriate drive with the label facing upwards and towards you.
- From the Windows Program Manager open the Main Program group, if it is closed, by double-clicking on the icon, then double-click on the File Manager Icon.
- Click once on Disk on the File Manager Menu Bar.
- When a drop-down menu appears, click once on Format Disk. The Format Disk dialogue box illustrated below will appear. Now follow the six instructions below.

**Figure A3.2** The 'Format disk' dialog box

❶ Place the cursor in the 'Label' box and click once then type a name to label your disk, for example, MYWORKDISK.

❷ If you want to format your disk at 720K or 360K, then click once on the down arrow in the 'Capacity' box, for an extended list, and click once on 720K or 360K.

❸ If you want to format your disk in drive B, then click once on the down arrow in the 'Disk In' box and click once on drive B.

❹ Click once on OK

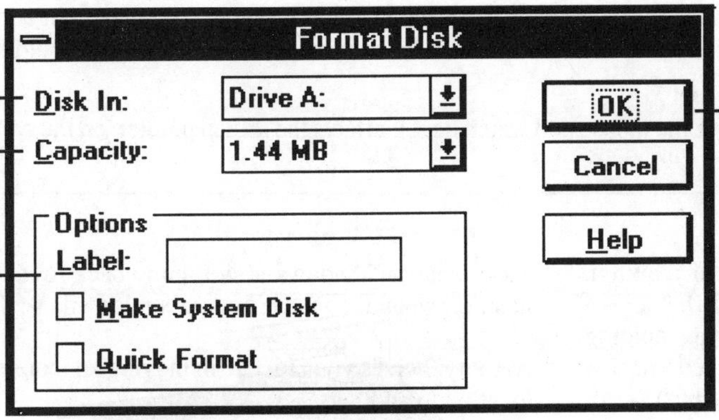

Format Disk
Disk In: Drive A:
Capacity: 1.44 MB
Options
Label:
Make System Disk
Quick Format
OK
Cancel
Help

❺ When the confirmation box appears choose YES to start the formatting process.

❻ When the disk is formatted you will be asked if you want to format another disk. Respond accordingly by clicking on the YES or NO button.

- If you want to make a system disk click once in the 'Make System Disk' box.
- If you are formatting a disk that has been formatted before you can click on the 'Quick Format' box, to format the disk quickly.

# APPENDIX 4
# Getting acquainted with Windows 3.1

### The input device

As already stated in Unit 8, with Windows some commands can only be issued with a mouse. If you have never used a mouse before, you might have some difficulties initially. With practice you are bound to improve your skill.

To remind you, the way to use the mouse is to hold it in the hand. The pointer is the arrow on the screen. It is controlled by the mouse. Sliding the mouse on a flat surface in the desired direction and pressing the mouse button are the only two actions involved in the basic skills of **pointing**, **clicking** and **dragging**.

An icon is selected on the screen by pointing to it and then pressing or clicking the mouse button. (Usually the left button.) All the activities below are designed to give you practice using the mouse.

## GLOSSARY OF TERMS 27

**Pointing** means placing the mouse pointer over a specific item or area on the screen.

**Clicking** means quickly pressing and releasing the mouse button in one non-stop action.

**Double click** means pressing and releasing the mouse button twice in rapid succession.

**Dragging** means pressing the mouse button and holding it down while moving the mouse. This technique is used to select text on the screen or move items from one place to another.

### ACTIVITY 1 – Using a mouse

If you have not already done so, switch on your computer and start Windows. Compare the screen on your computer with that of figures 8.1, 8.2 and 8.3 (*see* Unit 8). Even if your screen looks somewhat different you should see the screen pointer.

For the purpose of this exercise, simply move the mouse and watch how it affects the screen pointer on the computer screen.

### Moving icons

Icons can be moved to a different location if required. This is done by moving the mouse until the screen pointer is directly over it, then while pressing and holding the left button on the mouse. The icon is dragged to a new location. If an icon is moved to a position which is not acceptable to Windows, it will jump back to its original position when the mouse button is released.

Activity 2 gives you practice in moving an icon from one location to another.

### ACTIVITY 2 – Dragging an icon from one location to another

Using the mouse:

1. Move the pointer to an icon on the screen.
2. Press and hold down the left mouse button.
3. Move the icon to another location.
4. Release the mouse button to drop the icon in this new location.

## Opening and closing a Program Group

To open or close a Program Group icon is very simple. (For a reminder of group icons *see* Figure 8.1.) It is just a matter of pointing and clicking. An icon is successfully activitated when a sand-timer (Fig. A4.1)appears on the screen. Try the following activities.

**Figure A4.1** The sand-timer cursor

### ACTIVITY 3 – Opening a Program Group

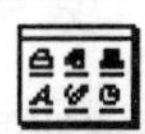


Locate a Program Group icon on the Program Manager window on your machine and open that group.

To open the Program Group:

1. Move the mouse to direct the screen pointer to a program group icon on the screen.
2. Double click on the left mouse button.

### ACTIVITY 4 – Closing a Program Group window

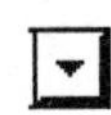

To close the Program Group window:

1. Move the mouse to direct the screen pointer to the down arrow on the TOP righthand corner of the window of that group which you have just opened.
2. Click once on the left mouse button.

### ACTIVITY 5 – Practice dragging and dropping using the mouse

Open the Program Group labelled Games. Double-click on the Solitaire icon. Have a game or two. This will help you develop your skill in handling the mouse.

## Practice

How did you get on with the above activties? Remember nothing comes without effort and practice.

### ACTIVITY 6 – Demonstration on how to use the mouse and work with Windows

Windows version 3.1 offers a computer tutorial on Windows. If you need to learn how to use the mouse or you need to brush up on your mouse skills, you should find the program helpful. To access the computer tutorial, you must first start Windows. When the Program Manager window appears, across the top you will find a series of menu options:

File, Options, Window, Help.

Move the mouse and direct the screen pointer over the Help menu. Click the left button of the mouse once. An expanded menu list will appear. Direct the screen pointer over the Windows Tutorial and once again click the left button of the mouse. The tutorial should start. Just follow the on-screen instructions.

# APPENDIX 5
# A guide to using MS-DOS commands

The assumption is that you are using a computer with a hard disk and at least one floppy disk drive. Boot up the computer then start Exercise 1.

**Important:** please type the commands exactly or they will not work. If you receive an error message after you have typed a command, check your entry.

**Exercise 1**
Boot up the computer. When you see the DOS prompt (C:\>) type the commands below exactly and see their effects.

| | |
|---|---|
| DIR | DIR tells DOS to display the content of the directory on the C drive.<br>At the DOS prompt type:<br>**DIR** then press **ENTER** |
| DIR/P | If the disk contains a substantial number of files, they will zoom up the screen faster than the eye can read them. You can stop the scrolling by telling DOS to pause when the screen is full.<br>At the DOS prompt type:<br>**DIR/P** then press **ENTER** |
| DIR/W | To tell DOS to produce a list using the full width of the screen you can use the command DIR/W.<br>At the DOS prompt type:<br>**DIR/W** then press **ENTER** |

| | |
|---|---|
| CLS | You can tell DOS to clear the screen leaving only the C:/> prompt.<br>At the DOS prompt type:<br>**CLS** then press **ENTER** |

| | |
|---|---|
| TYPE | If you want a text file such as AUTOEXEC.BAT to be displayed on the screen you can use the TYPE command.<br>At the DOS prompt type:<br>**TYPE AUTOEXEC.BAT** then press **ENTER** |
| >PRN | If you have a printer connected to the computer, switch it on. You can then print the result of the TYPE command.<br>At the DOS prompt type:<br>**TYPE AUTOEXEC.BAT >PRN** then press **ENTER** |

**Exercise 2**
At the DOS prompt (C:\>) type the commands below and follow the instructions on the screen.

| | |
|---|---|
| HELP | DOS has many more commands. You can tell DOS to show them to you by typing the command HELP.<br>At the DOS prompt type:<br>**HELP** then press **ENTER** |
| HELP MD | You can ask DOS for more explanation of specific commands. Suppose you want more information on how to make a directory.<br>At the DOS prompt type:<br>**HELP MD** then press **ENTER** |
| | Did you understand anything? What a load of gibberish, I hear you say. So much for user friendliness. |

**Exercise 3**
At the DOS prompt (C:\>) type the following commands.

| | |
|---|---|
| TREE | You can ask DOS to display the directory tree on the screen.<br>At the DOS prompt type:<br>**TREE** then press **ENTER** |
| MD or MKDIR | You can tell DOS to add a new directory to the tree. Suppose you want to add a directory called ZOO.<br>At the DOS prompt type:<br>**MD ZOO** then press **ENTER** |
| | *If you now type TREE you will be able to see the directory ZOO at the end of the DOS tree.* |
| RD or RMDIR | You can instruct DOS to remove a directory from the DOS tree. Suppose you now want to remove the directory called ZOO that you have just created above.<br>At the DOS prompt type:<br>**RD ZOO** then press **ENTER** |
| | *If you now type TREE you will be able to see if the directory ZOO has really been removed from the DOS tree.* |

There are many more DOS commands that are worth exploring. **You should only try them under guidance.**

As pointed out in Unit 7, a filename can have up to eight characters plus an extension name of up to three characters. However, when choosing names for files that you have created for your documents or programs, you should avoid using the following names because they are names of commands or files in DOS.

| | |
|---|---|
| APPEND | Allows programs to open data files in specified directories as if they were in the current directory. |
| ASSIGN | Assigns a drive letter to a different drive. |
| ATTRIB | Displays or changes the attributes of selected files in a directory. |
| BACKUP | Backs up one or more files from one disk to another. |
| BREAK | Sets or clears extended CTRL+C checking. |
| CALL | Calls one batch program from another. |
| CD or CHDIR | Displays the name of or changes the current directory. |
| CHCP | Displays or changes the current code page for the command processor COMMAND.COM. |
| CHKDSK | Scans the disk in the specified drive and checks it for errors then displays a report. |
| CHKDSK /f | Fixes broken chains on disk. |
| COMMAND | Starts a new instance of the MS-DOS command interpreter. |
| COMP | Compares the contents of two files or sets of files. |
| COPY | Copies one or more files to another location. |
| CTTY | Lets you change the device from which you issue commands. |
| DATE | Displays or sets the date. |
| DEBUG | Runs Debug, a tool for writing and editing small programs. |
| DEL or ERASE | Deletes or erases one or more files. |
| DISKCOMP | Compares the contents of two floppy disks. |
| DISKCOPY | Copies the contents of one floppy disk in the source drive to a formatted or unformatted floppy disk in a target drive. |
| DOSKEY | Edits command lines, recalls MS-DOS commands and creates macros. |
| DOSSHELL | Starts MS-DOS Shell. |
| ECHO | Displays messages or turns command echoing on or off. |
| EDIT | Starts MS-DOS Editor, which creates and changes ASCII files. |
| EDLIN | Starts Edlin, a line-oriented text editor. |
| EMM386 | Turns on or off EMM386 expanded memory support. |
| EXE2BIN | Converts .EXE (executable) files to binary format. |
| EXIT | Exits or quits the COMMAND.COM program (command interpreter) and returns to a previous level if one exists. |
| EXPAND | Expands one or more compressed files. |
| FASTOPEN | Decreases the amount of time needed to open frequently used files and directories. |
| FC | Compares two files or sets of files and displays the differences between them. |
| FDISK | Configures a hard disk for use with MS-DOS. |
| FIND | Searches for a text string in a file or files. |
| FOR | Runs a specified command for each file in a set of files. |
| FORMAT | Formats a disk for use with MS-DOS. |
| GOTO | Directs MS-DOS to a labelled line in a batch program. |
| GRAFTABL | Enables MS-DOS to display an extended character set in graphics mode. |
| GRAPHICS | Lets you print a graphics display screen on a printer when you are using a colour or graphics monitor adapter. |
| HELP | Provides information on MS-DOS commands. |
| IF | Performs conditional processing in batch programs. |
| JOIN | Joins a disk drive to a directory on another drive. |

| | |
|---|---|
| KEYB | Configures a keyboard for a specific language. |
| LABEL | Creates or deletes the volume label of a disk. |
| LH | Loads a program into the upper memory area. |
| LOADFIX | Loads a program above the first 64 Kb of memory and runs the program. |
| LOADHIGH | Loads a program into the upper memory area. |
| MEM | Displays the amount of used and free memory in your system. |
| MIRROR | Records information about one or more disks. |
| MODE | Configures a system device. |
| MORE | Displays output one screen at a time. |
| NLSFUNC | Loads country-specific information. |
| PATH | Displays or sets a search path for files. |
| PAUSE | Suspends processing of a batch file and displays a message. |
| PRINT | Prints a text file while you are using other MS-DOS commands. |
| PROMPT | Changes the MS-DOS command prompt. |
| QBASIC | Starts the MS-DOS QBasic programming environment. |
| RECOVER | Recovers readable information from a bad or defective disk. |
| REM | Records comments (remarks) in batch files or CONFIG.SYS. |
| REN or RENAME | Renames a file or files. |
| REPLACE | Replaces files. |
| RESTORE | Restores files that were backed up using the BACKUP command. |
| SET | Displays or removes MS-DOS environment variables. |
| SETVER | Sets the version number that MS-DOS reports to a program. |
| SHARE | Installs file-sharing and locking capabilities on your hard disk. |
| SHIFT | Shifts the position of replaceable parameters in batch files. |
| SORT | Sorts input. |
| SUBST | Associates a path with a drive letter. |
| SYS | Copies MS-DOS system files and the command interpreter to a disk you specify. |
| TIME | Displays or sets the system time. |
| UNDELETE | Recovers files which have been deleted. |
| UNFORMAT | Restores a disk erased by the FORMAT command or restructured by the RECOVER command. |
| VER | Displays the MS-DOS version. |
| VERIFY | Tells MS-DOS whether to verify that your files are written correctly to a disk. |
| VOL | Displays a disk volume label and serial number. |
| XCOPY | Copies files (except hidden and system files) and directory trees. |

# Appendix 6
# A step-by-step guide to using Minitab

There are many statistics packages available, some more sophisticated than others. ABSTAT, SPSS and Minitab are examples of such programs.

ABSTAT contains a variety of parametric and nonparametric statistical tests and will run on a personal computer (PC).

SPSS (Statistical Package for the Social Sciences) is available for use on mainframe (e.g. the VAX) and will also run on PCs. SPSS is the most frequently used statistical package. It can be used to conduce numerous parametric and nonparametric analyses and to generate a multitude of tables, charts and graphs.

Minitab is a particularly accessible statistics package, still used by many institutions in the pursuit of research. It provides a good introduction to the use of stats packages and, having come to grips with it, you will find it easier to move on to other packages if you so wish. It too can produce charts and graphs. There is a DOS and a Windows version. The DOS version is much more suitable for beginners, especially if you are not familiar with using Windows. The following exercises are intended to help you get started with Minitab (DOS version release 7.2) **and should be done in the sequence laid out.**

The following assumptions have been made:

- that the computer or network you are using has got Minitab Release 7.2 installed on it;
- that you know how to switch on a computer;
- that you are familiar with the terms C prompt (on a stand-alone system) or N prompt (on a network), drives A, B, C or N and directory;
- that you are familiar with MS-DOS commands, particularly CD or CHDIR;
- that you know and understand the concept of a spreadsheet.

If these are not correct, you should first read Section 3.4 and/or Unit 7. You should also complete the exercises in Unit 7 before attempting to activate Minitab.

---

**ACTIVITY 1 – Activating Minitab**

Before you can work with Minitab the program needs to be activated. To activate the program you first need to instruct the computer to move to the directory where Minitab is stored.

- To move to the directory where Minitab is normally stored, type the following after the C:\> prompt
  **CD MINITAB**

- If you have not already done so, now press the RETURN or ENTER key once. On your screen you should now see the following:
  **C:\MINITAB>**

- To activate Minitab, you simply type the following then press RETURN.
  **MINITAB**

The screen will change and you should see a screen as shown in Figure A6.1 (note: the wording may not match exactly).

- If you now press any key the screen will change again to display the screen shown in Figure A6.2.
- Minitab is now ready for you to use. Please complete the following activities.

**MINITAB**

Data Analysis Software
Release 7.2 -- Standard Version
Copyright (C) Minitab, Inc. 1989

This software is licensed to:

(name of the company of person owning the software)
Serial # .........

You may use MINITAB under the terms of the License Agreement enclosed with this program; please read it. This License entitles: a) one user to run this copy of MINITAB on any number of computers; b) more than one user to run this copy of MINITAB on a single computer, BUT it is a violation of the License to run this copy of MINITAB on more than one computer simultaneously. Government users see HELP FGU

Press any key to continue.

**Figure A6.1** Minitab opening screen

MINITAB Release 7.2 *** COPYRIGHT - Minitab, Inc. 1989
Standard Version *** Storage Available: 16179
JAN. 13, 1994

Use the ESCape key to toggle between Minitab and Data Editor

MTB>

**Figure A6.2** A Minitab screen

**ACTIVITY 2 – Minitab worksheet (data editor)**

You can toggle between Minitab and the Minitab worksheet by simply pressing the escape (ESC) key on the keyboard. Do this:

- Press the ESC key again and again. See what happens.

With each press you should find yourself either looking at the WORKSHEET or at the Minitab screen.

**ACTIVITY 3 – The worksheet**

- If you have not already done so, press the ESC key to display the Minitab worksheet.
  As you can see, it looks just like a spreadsheet, with columns and rows. The columns are labelled with the letter C followed by a number, while the rows are simply numbered. Minitab offers 99 columns and 999 rows. If you inspect the worksheet on the screen you will note that in the left-hand corner (column C1, row 1) there is a single box which is highlighted. This box indicates where the cursor is. To move the cursor from one cell to another simply press the arrow pointing in the direction you want to go. For example, if you want to move to the right, you press this arrow:➡. To move down one cell you press this arrow: ⬇, and so on.

Familiarize yourself with the worksheet by moving around it in any direction, starting with ➡

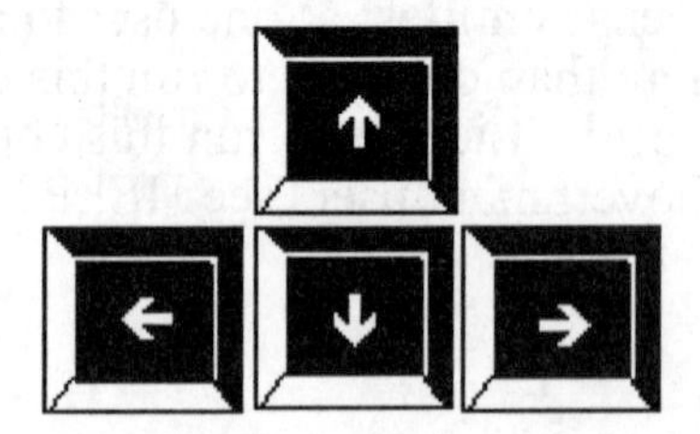

**Figure A6.3** The arrow keys

**ACTIVITY 4 – Labelling the columns in your worksheet**

All the columns can be labelled. For our purpose, we are going to label columns C1 to C4 with the following names: age, sex, cigbrand, numsmoke. To do this do the following.

- If the cursor is not already there, move it to column C1, row 1.
- Now press the up arrow ⬆ once. The highlighted cursor jumps above C1.
- Type your first label: age.
- Press the RETURN or ENTER key. The cursor moves to above C2.
- Type sex in C2, cigbrand in C3 and numsmoke in C4.

**Help:** If you have inadvertently misspelt a label, simply return the cursor to the appropriate box, and type the correct label. You use the same tactic with data that have been wrongly typed.

## ACTIVITY 5 – Entering data directly into the worksheet

There are two ways to enter data in Minitab. Data can be retrieved from a file previously stored on disk or typed in by hand using the keyboard. To enter data directly into the worksheet do this:

- Ensure the cursor is in column C1. row 1.

Type the following data in the appropriate columns.

| | *age* C1 | *sex* C2 | *cigbrand* C3 | *numsmoke* C4 |
|---|---|---|---|---|
| 1 | 23 | 0 | 1 | 20 |
| 2 | 34 | 0 | 1 | 50 |
| 3 | 45 | 1 | 2 | 10 |
| 4 | 21 | 0 | 3 | 60 |
| 5 | 30 | 1 | 2 | 40 |
| 6 | 23 | 1 | 1 | 40 |
| 7 | 36 | 0 | 2 | 60 |
| 8 | 44 | 0 | 1 | 30 |
| 9 | 40 | 1 | 2 | 50 |
| 10 | 25 | 1 | 2 | 40 |

**Help:** When you press the RETURN/ENTER key after data entry, the cursor will automatically move to the next column. When you get to C4, use the left arrow ← to bring the cursor back to column C1, row 1. Then use the down arrow↓ to move the cursor to column C1, row 2.

**Hint:** To enter data down a single column you follow each entry by pressing the down arrow instead of RETURN/ENTER.

## ACTIVITY 6 – Saving your worksheet to disk

Typically, files stored using Minitab are followed by the suffix .MTW. The suffix is added automatically by the program. To save the worksheet you typed in Activity 5 do this:

- Press ESC to leave the Minitab worksheet.

The screen will change and among other things you should now see:

**MTB >**

We are going to name our worksheet: 'mydata'. Now to save the worksheet to drive C (if you are using a stand-alone system with a hard disk) do this:

- Type the following after the MTB > prompt:

**SAVE 'MYDATA'**

If you have followed the above instructions correctly you should see the following on the screen:
Worksheet saved into file: mydata.MTW

**Help:** if you have made a mistake (for example, you forgot to enclose the filename in quotation marks), Minitab will display an appropriate error message and save the worksheet in a file called MINITAB.MTW. I suggest you try saving the worksheet again using the above instructions and filename so that you can do Activity 8.

**ACTIVITY 7 – Quitting Minitab**

When you have finished using Minitab, you simply type 'stop' after the prompt to exit from the application and return to the Minitab directory. Do this:

- After the Minitab prompt type:

**STOP**

- Press the RETURN key.

```
*** Minitab Release 7.2 *** Minitab, Inc. ***
Storage available 161179

C:\MINITAB>
```

**ACTIVITY 8 – Retrieving a Minitab worksheet**

If you have done Activity 7 as instructed you will need to reactivate Minitab before we can continue. So do this:

- Reactivate Minitab (see Activity 1, if necessary).
- Type the following command after the Minitab prompt:

**MTB > retrieve 'mydata'**

- Press the RETURN key.

Displayed on the screen beneath MTB>retrieve 'mydata' you should see the following:

**WORKSHEET SAVED (date)**
**Worksheet retrieved from file: mydata.MTW**
**MTB>**

- Press the ESC key.

Displayed on the screen should be the Minitab worksheet containing the data entered in Activity 5.

**ACTIVITY 9 – Using Minitab help**

There is a help facility that helps you learn about Minitab. To activate the help facility type 'help' after the Minitab prompt, like so:

**MTB > help**

Do not forget to press the RETURN key after you have typed 'help'. You should now be able to use Minitab to analyse your data by following the instructions on the screen. If you encounter difficulties, refer to the manual.

# APPENDIX 7
# Checklist for evaluating application software

This checklist is intended as a diagnostic tool for assessing the usefulness of a particularly application software package. Any negative answer indicates an area that should be given full consideration when deciding whether or not to accept the software in its current state. This checklist is also useful, of course, as a guide for evaluating software developed by in-house programmer(s).

## CHECKLIST

| | | Yes | No |
|---|---|---|---|
| **USER FRIENDLINESS** | | | |
| 1 | Does the user clearly know when the computer is waiting for an input? | | |
| 2 | Does the user know what kind of input the program expects? | | |
| 3 | Does the program run without breaking down? | | |
| 4 | Is the screen display easy to read and understand? | | |
| 5 | Can the user correct his/her inputs? | | |
| 6 | Does the software offer audible warning when the user's input is incorrect? | | |
| 7 | Does the software offer help after the user has responded incorrectly? | | |
| 8 | Can the user request on-screen help? | | |
| 9 | Can the user quit the program at any point? | | |
| 10 | Is the accompanying documentation concise and easy to understand? | | |
| 11 | Does the program remind the user to save data entered? | | |
| 12 | Does the program have automatic backup facility? | | |
| 13 | Does the program have an undelete facility? | | |
| **EQUIPMENT** | | | |
| 14 | Can the software be run on your existing equipment or network? | | |
| 15 | Does your equipment have the required amount of memory to run the software? | | |
| 16 | Does your equipment have the required peripherals to use the software? | | |
| **STRUCTURE AND MANAGEMENT** | | | |
| 17 | Has the program got a password facility? | | |
| 18 | Does the program protect data already entered in the event of a sudden electrical failure? | | |
| 19 | Will the program interfere with other applications already installed in the computer? | | |
| 20 | Does the program allow for import and export of data and/or graphics? | | |
| **GENERAL** | | | |
| 21 | Is the program good value for money? | | |
| 22 | Is there a competing program that offers better value for money? | | |
| 23 | Is the program easy to learn? | | |
| 24 | Are you allowed to make a backup copy of the program? | | |
| 25 | Will you be receiving updates and how much extra will you need to pay? | | |
| 26 | What after-sale support is available? | | |
| 27 | What is the licensing policy? | | |
| 28 | Is there any staff training being offered with the program? | | |

# APPENDIX 8
# Checklist for evaluating educational software

Differentiating good educational software from bad is not very easy for practising nurses or nurse educators who have not experienced educational computing as a part of general or professional education. However, with the growing acceptance of computers in clinical settings (Scarpa *et al*., 1992; Chellen, 1994), software needs to be properly assessed before it is purchased, especially given the fact that educational software does not always meet the standards and specifications of the nursing departments within a particular institution.

Purchasing software that has not been properly evaluated can be costly. To assist nurse educators and practitioners in making informed, effective and competent decisions before purchasing educational software, several checklists and evaluation tools have been published, by Hudgings and Meehan (1984), Hannafin and Peck (1988) and Bolwell (1991), to name but a few. The checklist below is an adaptation of these so that it is uniquely applicable to clinical settings.

---

Note for evaluator(s): any negative answer indicates an area that should be given full consideration when deciding whether or not to accept the software.

| **EQUIPMENT** | **Yes** | **No** |
|---|---|---|
| Can the software be run on your existing equipment? | | |
| Does your equipment have the required peripherals to use the software? | | |
| Does your equipment have the required amount of memory to run the software? | | |
| Can the software be run on network as well as stand-alone systems? | | |
| **OBJECTIVES AND CONTENTS** | | |
| Are the learning objectives clearly stated? | | |
| Is the material relevant? | | |
| Is the material current? | | |
| Is the material free from content errors? | | |
| Is the language used clear and understandable? | | |
| Can the material be used to support other teaching and learning activities? | | |
| Is the material appropriate to the target group? | | |
| Is the user input appropriate to the objectives? | | |
| **STRUCTURE AND MANAGEMENT** | | |
| Does the program move the student step by step? | | |
| Does the material encourage problem solving or creative responses? | | |
| Does the program track individual performance? | | |
| Does the program allow the student/teacher to select the level of difficulty? | | |
| Does the program summarize/comment on the student's performance during or at the end of the run? | | |
| Does the program have a password facility for the teacher? | | |

| **VISUAL APPEAL** | **Yes** | **No** |
|---|---|---|
| Does the program make effective use of : | | |
| highlighted text? | | |
| colour? | | |
| sound/audio? | | |
| still graphics and animations? | | |
| **USER FRIENDLINESS** | | |
| Does the user clearly know when the computer is waiting for an input? | | |
| Does the user know what kind of input the program expects? | | |
| Does the program run without breaking down? | | |
| Is the screen display easy to read and understand? | | |
| Can the user correct his or her inputs? | | |
| Does the software offer help or provide a correct answer after the user has responded incorrectly? | | |
| Does the software offer an audible warning when the user's input is incorrect? | | |
| Can the user request on-screen help? | | |
| Can the user quit the program at any point? | | |
| Is the accompanying documentation concise and easy to understand? | | |
| **GENERAL** | | |
| Is the program good value for money? | | |
| Is there a competing program that offers better value for money? | | |
| What is the manufacturer's: | | |
| backup policy? | | |
| updates policy? | | |
| after sale support? | | |
| site licensing policy? | | |

# APPENDIX 9
# A short guide to the Cumulative Index to Nursing and Allied Health Literature (CINAHL)

**CINAHL** is a compact disk designed specifically to meet the information needs of nurses and allied health professionals. It is the database equivalent to printed CINAHL. This bibliographic database was started in 1983 and is updated bi-monthly. It contains more than 130,000 records from more than 500 English-language journals, books, pamphlets dissertations and educational software in nursing and allied health professions. Records on the CINAHL CD-ROM are divided into several fields, including title, authors, publisher, publication year, abstract and many more. All the commands used to operate the system appear at the bottom of the screen.

---

## Searching CINAHL

Once you have selected CINAHL from the screen menu, by pressing the function key labelled F10, all the commands used to operate the system will appear at the bottom of the screen.The first letter of each command is highlighted. You simply press the letter indicated to operate the command.

## Search by author

- Select FIND or INDEX commands.
- Type in the surname and (if known) the initial(s), e.g. Carter-BE.
- Now press the RETURN key.

## Searching by subject

If you want to scan the database for information on particular subjects you should use FIND, INDEX or THESAURUS.

- THESAURUS and INDEX display subject terms used by the database, with associated topical subheadings and age categories.
- FIND is used for free text searching, i.e. searching for terms not located in the THESAURUS, and for combining terms and search sets together. To combine terms the following operators can be used: AND, OR, NOT. For example, to find two terms in the same record you can type:

**health AND alcohol**

To find either term you can type:

**health OR alcohol**

To search for one record and exclude another you can type:

**health NOT alcohol**

- Select the FIND command.
- Type the subject you want, for example: **computers AND nursing**
- Now press the RETURN key.

# REVISION TEST

**Instructions:** Consolidate your knowledge by answering the following questions. You can check your answers by going back to the text.

| For answers refer to: | | |
|---|---|---|
| Section 1.1 | **Q1** | What is a computer? |
| Section 2.5 | **Q2** | List fourteen precautions that should be taken when handling a floppy disk. |
| Section 3.3 | **Q3** | What is a database application program? |
| Unit 4 | **Q4** | List the five basic components of a computer. |
| Facts 5 | **Q5** | What does the acronym IBM stand for? |
| Section 6.2 | **Q6** | List the eight internationally agreed principles relating to personal data. |
| Section 7.3 | **Q7** | How many characters can a filename extension have using MS-DOS? |
| Section 7.1 | **Q8** | What is the role of the operating system? |
| Section 8.2 | **Q9** | What is an icon? |
| Facts 25 | **Q10** | What does FORTRAN stand for? |
| Unit 11 | **Q11** | Outline six limitations of computers. |
| Unit 1 | **Q12** | What is meant by the following terms:<br>(a) hardware<br>(b) software<br>(c) MS-DOS<br>(d) application programs<br>(e) CPU |
| Unit 2 | **Q13** | List four devices that can be connected to a computer. |
| Section 3.3 | **Q14** | State two advantages and two disadvantages of a database system in the ward situation. |
| Section 4.1 | **Q15** | Name six input devices. |
| Section 5.3 | **Q16** | What is the typical internal memory capacity of a microcomputer? |
| Section 6.2 | **Q17** | What is the role of the Data Protection Registrar? |
| Section 7.3 | **Q18** | Complete the following blanks. The first floppy disk drive on a stand-alone system is usually referred to as ___ and the second as ___. |
| Section 8.2 | **Q19** | What device controls the screen pointer in Windows? |
| Facts 24 | **Q20** | What is a screen pointer? |

| Reference | | Question |
|---|---|---|
| Section 10.3 | **Q21** | List five research activities that can be facilitated by computers. |
| Section 11.1 | **Q22** | Give two ways of minimizing the risk of losing data from the computer in the event of electrical failure. |
| Unit 5 | **Q23** | What is meant by a computer system? List three types. |
| Facts 2 | **Q24** | List eight features that ought to be taken into account when selecting a printer. |
| Section 2.5 | **Q25** | State why it is necessary to format a new disk. |
| Section 3.1 | **Q26** | Give two reasons for saving work done on a word processor on to storage media such as disks or tapes. |
| Section 5.1 | **Q27** | Which type of computer is the most powerful? |
| Section 6.2 | **Q28** | What are the implications of the Data Protection Act for health professionals? |
| Section 7.5 | **Q29** | What is the difference between a program file and a data file? |
| Section 8.2 | **Q30** | Label (a) and (b) in the diagram below. |
| Section 8.2 | **Q31** | What does GUI stand for? |
| Table 10.1 | **Q32** | List five databases that are useful for research in nursing. |
| Unit 11 | **Q33** | What is the name given to the semiconducting element from which computer chips are made? |
| Section 1.2 | **Q34** | List the three pieces of hardware that make up a computer system. |
| Section 2.3 | **Q35** | How does a fax-modem differ from a fax machine? |
| Section 3.4 | **Q36** | List four possible uses for a spreadsheet in clinical settings. |
| Sections 4.3 and 4.4 | **Q37** | Explain the following types of memory:<br>(a) RAM<br>(b) ROM<br>(c) PROM<br>(d) EPROM |
| Section 5.1 | **Q38** | What is the typical RAM of a mainframe computer? |
| Section 6.3 | **Q39** | How can unauthorized personnel be prevented from gaining access to personal data kept in a computer? |
| Facts 22 | **Q40** | What are UNIX and OS/2? |
| Section 9.2 | **Q41** | What is a query language? |
| Section 10.2 | **Q42** | What is meant by input errors and programming errors? |
| Activity 1 | **Q43** | List the areas of nursing where computers cannot outsmart humans. |

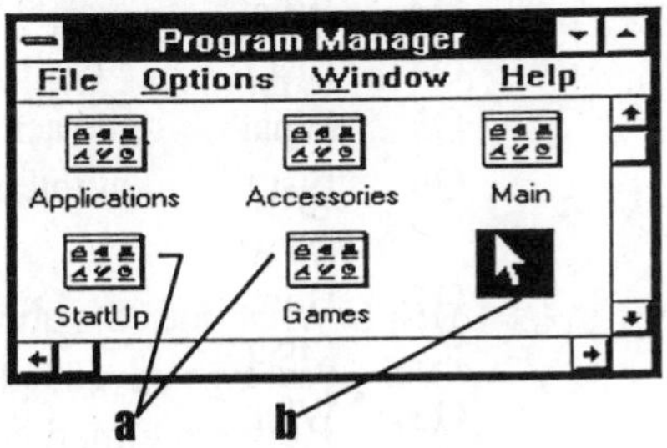

| Reference | Question | |
|---|---|---|
| Facts 22 | **Q44** | List three types of disk operating system. |
| Section 2.5 | **Q45** | Differentiate between a floppy disk and a hard disk. |
| Section 3.5 | **Q46** | What do you understand by e-mail? |
| Section 4.1 | **Q47** | How can a bar code system be used in clinical areas? |
| Section 5.3 | **Q48** | Laptop computers cannot be fitted with a modem because they are too small. True or false? |
| Section 6.4 | **Q49** | What is the aim of the Health and Safety Regulations of 1992 with regard to VDUs? |
| Glossary 25 | **Q50** | What is the name of this object? |
| Section 8.2 | **Q51** | What is special about the StartUp Program Group? |
| Facts 25 | **Q52** | Name seven high-level computer languages. |
| Facts 26 | **Q53** | What arithmetic operation is represented by each of these symbols?<br>(a) <<br>(b) ><br>(c) * |
| Glossary 1 | **Q54** | What does the abbreviation VDU stand for? |
| Table 3.3 | **Q55** | List two advantages and two disadvantages of e-mail. |
| Section 3.5 | **Q56** | How can e-mail be used by practitioners to enhance care? |
| Section 6.3 | **Q57** | Bugs in DOS itself are one of the commonest causes of data loss. What is meant by the term 'bug' here? |
| Section 5.3 | **Q58** | What type of screen would you expect to find on a laptop? |
| Section 6.4 | **Q59** | List the obligations of employers under the Health and Safety Regulations 1992 with regard to VDUs. |
| Appendix 5 | **Q60** | DIR is short for what? |
| Section 8.2 | **Q61** | Describe how you select an icon in Windows using the mouse. |
| Section 9.2 | **Q62** | Explain what is meant by a low-level computer language. |
| Section 10.3 | **Q63** | Name two statistical packages available for computer analysis of nursing data. |
| Glossary 1 | **Q64** | Give two other names for the VDU. |
| Unit 3 | **Q65** | List five functions of a computer. |
| Section 3.5 | **Q66** | What is the meaning of LAN and WAN and how do they differ? |
| Section 4.3 | **Q67** | What is meant by the following terms:<br>(a) input<br>(b) ASCII<br>(c) byte<br>(d) interface<br>(e) menu |
| Section 6.2 | **Q68** | What are the obligations of data users with regard to personal data? |

| Reference | | Question |
|---|---|---|
| Table 6.2 | **Q69** | List six health problems which may result from prolonged use of VDUs. |
| Appendix 5 | **Q70** | What would you use the following DOS programs for?<br>(a) CHKDSK.EXE<br>(b) DISKCOPY.EXE |
| Unit 8 | **Q71** | What is Windows? |
| Facts 24 | **Q72** | Name nine common errors made by users when entering commands into a computer. |
| Section 10.3 | **Q73** | How can WordPerfect be used in qualitative analysis of data? |
| Unit 1 Activity 1 | **Q74** | What types of computers are in use in health care settings? |
| Section 3.1 | **Q75** | List two possible uses of a word processor in clinical settings. |
| Section 10.3 | **Q76** | Name one statistical package that can be used to analyse nursing data. |
| Section 5.1 | **Q77** | What is a mainframe computer? |
| Section 6.2 | **Q78** | What is meant by the following terms?<br>(a) data user<br>(b) data subject<br>(c) computer bureau<br>(d) personal data |
| Table 6.2 | **Q79** | List four actions that an employee can take to minimize the risk of ill-health from the use of VDUs. |
| Appendix 5 | **Q80** | What would you use the following DOS commands for?<br>CD<br>DIR<br>MD<br>RD |
| Unit 8 | **Q81** | What is WIMP? |
| Facts 24 | **Q82** | What does the word BASIC stand for? |
| Unit 10 | **Q83** | A microcomputer cannot be used for data analysis because it does not have enough memory. True or false? |
| Unit 1 and Section 3.8 | **Q84** | What software packages are health professionals using to manage health care? |
| Table 3.1 | **Q85** | What are the advantages of a word processor over a typewriter? |
| Section 3.7 | **Q86** | What is an expert system? |
| Unit 5 | **Q87** | What is the generic name of the smallest computer in common use? |
| Section 6.2 | **Q88** | What are the obligations of computer bureaux with regard to personal data? |
| Section 7.3 | **Q89** | How many characters can a filename have using MS-DOS? |
| Section 7.3 | **Q90** | State the purpose of a directory and subdirectory. |
| Section 8.2 | **Q91** | What is the difference between 'windows' and 'Windows'? |
| Facts 25 | **Q92** | What does COBOL stand for? |
| Facts 22 | **Q93** | List five types of operating system. |

Figure 2.4 — **Q94** What size of disk is this?

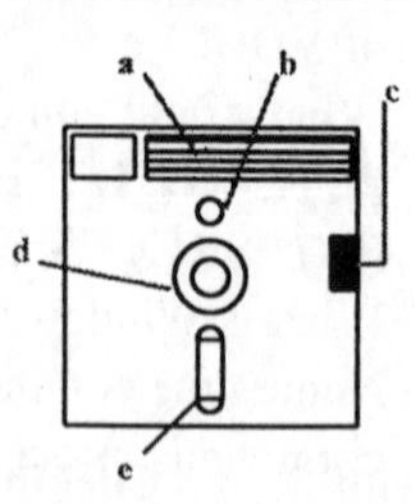


Figure 2.4 — **Q95** Identify the following in the above diagram:

(a) index hole
(b) hub
(c) window
(d) write protect notch
(e) label

Section 4.5 — **Q96** What is meant by output?

Section 4.5 — **Q97** Name two output devices.

Section 2.3 — **Q98** What are the following devices?

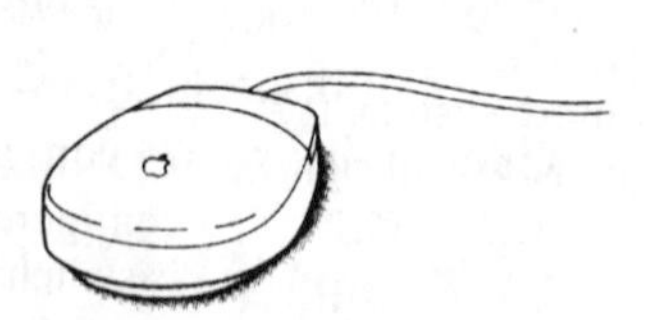

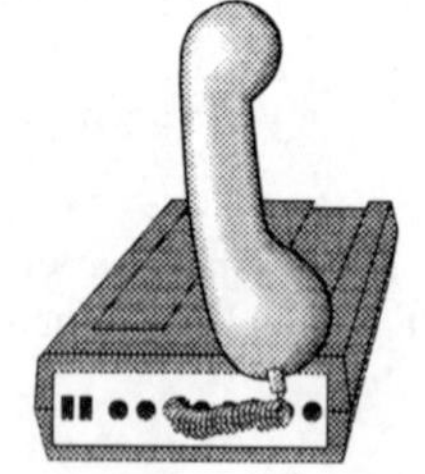

Sections 2.2 and 2.3 — **Q99** What are the two devices in Q98 used for?

Section 3.7 — **Q100** How can an expert system be used in clinical areas?

# GLOSSARY OF TERMS

**Accessories** are materials required for use with the computer.

**ALU** is an abbreviation of arithmetic logic unit. This is the part of the processor where the arithmetical, logical and other operations are carried out. These include arithmetic (such as add, subtract, multiply and divide), comparison (such as 'does selling price exceed cost?') and branch operations (which change the order of program instructions) and the movement of data.

**Application programs** are pre-written programs which contain specific instructions to enable the computer to carry out tasks such as word processing or accounting.

**ASCII.** The acronym for American Standard Code for Information Interchange, a widely used system for encoding letters, numerals, punctuation marks and signs as binary numbers.

**AUTOEXEC.BAT** is a file which contains instructions that will tell MS-DOS to carry out a particular task automatically when the computer is switched on.

**Automatically processed** in this context is taken to mean processing by use of computing equipment.

**Booting up** is the process of switching on the computer and loading the operating system into the RAM.

**Byte.** A sequence of bits, usually eight, treated as a unit for computation or storage.

**Bytes.** File sizes are measured in bytes. One byte is the amount of space it takes to store a character . A kilobyte (Kb) is 1024 bytes. A megabyte (Mb) is 1024 Kb.

**CD-ROM** is an abbreviation for Compact Disk-Read Only Memory. It is one type of optical storage media. The user can only retrieve the information stored on this type of disk, not store new material.

A **chip** is a collection of microscopic electrical circuits stamped on to a piece of silicon, made up of thousands of transistors and other electronic components.

**Clicking** means quickly pressing and releasing the mouse button in one non-stop action.

A **computer bureau** is an organization or individual that processes personal data for data users, or allows the user to process personal data on its equipment. An organization or individual may thus rank as a computer bureau (e.g. by providing back-up facilities for another data user) without actually being in business as a computer bureau as such.

A **computer** is a programmable machine that accepts, processes and displays information/data.

A **computer system** is a group of interacting parts that operate together to achieve a common end.

**CONFIG.SYS** is a file that contains instructions that configure various parts of MS-DOS when the computer is switched on.

The **CPU** – central processing unit – is the part of a computer that interprets and executes instructions. It is composed of an arithmetic logic chip, a control unit and a small amount of memory.

**Data** are raw facts and figures and for the purposes of the Data Protection Act this means any information stored in a machine which can be automatically processed.

A **database** can be described as a sophisticated electronic filing cabinet capable of sorting data in an organized manner. The data can be accessed quickly as desired.

A **data subject** is an individual to whom personal data relates.

**Data users** are organizations or individuals that control the contents and use of a collection of personal data processed, or intended to be processed, automatically.

**Desktop** is a term used to refer to a computer that is usually placed somewhere on a desk.

A **desktop publishing** application, also referred to as

DTP, is a sophisticated word processor. It offers greater control over the finished document.

A **directory** is a table of contents for a disk. It holds names of and information about the position of each file stored on the disk.

A **disk** is a round magnetized plate, usually made of plastic or metal, organized into concentric tracks and pie-slice shaped sectors for storing data. There are a number of different types of disk. See Section 2.5 for more information.

A **document** is a piece of work with a specific name, produced on a computer, which if stored can be retrieved immediately or at a later time.

**Double-clicking** means pressing and releasing the mouse button twice in rapid succession.

**Dragging** means pressing the mouse button and holding it down while moving the mouse. This technique is used to select text on the screen or move items from one place to another.

**Electronic mail** or **e-mail** is a relatively new concept in human communications. It allows people to send each other information, messages, notes, drawings, software and letters immediately without putting them to paper.

**EPROM** is short for erasable programmable read only memory. This is the same as PROM except that the information can be erased and the chip reprogrammed.

An **expert system** is a computer program which possesses knowledge rather than figures and words. The program must use logical reasoning procedures, allowing problems to be solved.

**Facsimile** or **fax** is different from e-mail. Messages, notes, drawings, listings of software and letters which have been prepared using a word processor have to be printed on to paper first. The paper containing the text/drawing is then fed into a fax machine. The machine takes a 'picture' of the text or drawing and transmits the picture to its destination via the telephone line. An ordinary fax machine can communicate with a computer with a fax-modem and vice versa.

**Field.** In the context of a database each title or subtitle on a record is referred to as a field (the term also refers to an area of a screen that is designated to hold a specified piece of information).

A **file** is a collection of related information, like the contents of a file folder in a desk drawer.

A **filename** is a unique name assigned to a file.

A **filename extension**, as the name suggests, is additional information attached to the filename, often describing the format of a file.

A **floppy disk** is a small flexible medium, usually magnetic, on which information is recorded for future use.

**Formatting** is the process of preparing a disk so that data can be stored upon it. A special program is used to carry out this process. Once a disk has been formatted it does not normally require formatting again.

A **gateway** is an interface, perhaps between networks, perhaps between a network and a major computer system, and usually involves both hardware and software.

**GIGO** is an acronym for garbage in, garbage out.

A **grammar checker** is a computer program which allows the user to check grammatical errors. The program will display suggestions, which you can ignore if you choose to.

**Hackers** are normally skilled programmers who invade systems and ferret out information on individual computer access codes through a process of trial and error.

A **hard disk** is an alternative to floppies. It has two or more rigid disks stacked on top of each other in a sealed case. It is much faster, and can store far more data, than a floppy disk.

**Hardware** is the physical or tangible apparatus of a computer system, i.e. all input and output devices.

**Icon** is the name given to certain graphic objects you see in the window, when Windows has been activated. They are used in conjunction with a cursor and pointer for selecting options from drop-down menus, or for running programs or tasks.

An **input device** is a piece of hardware for inputting information into the computer, e.g. keyboard, mouse.

**Input** is the information you provide to the computer.

**Interface** is used as both a noun and a verb. As a noun it means a two-way connection, and as a verb it means to cooperate or interconnect.

**JANET (Joint Academic Network)** is a government-funded computer network. It is designed to support UK academic and research communities, by providing access to other institution facilities (e.g. library catalogues, research banks, on-line conferences), and by allowing communication with members of those institutions via e-mail.

**LAN** refers to a system of interconnected PCs and other devices over a small area, typically within a few hundred yards, linked directly by cables. It is an abbreviation for local area network.

**Long haul network** is an alternative term for WAN.

**Magneto-optical** is a storage medium. Unlike CD-ROM or WORM, the content of the disk can be altered.

A **mainframe** is a large computer with a large amount of memory which has the ability to serve several users simultaneously.

A **menu** is a list of options from which the user can make a selection.

A **modem** is a device that enables data to be transmitted between computers, generally over telephone lines, but sometimes on fibre-optic cable or radio frequencies. It enables one computer to talk to another through translating (MOdulating) computer binary signals into telephone analogue signals and back again (DEModulating).

A **monitor** is a television-like output device for displaying data. Also referred to as a VDU (visual display unit).

**MS-DOS** is an abbreviation for Microsoft Disk Operating System. Several alternative operating systems are available.

**Network** is a general term used to describe the connection of compatible computers.

An **operating system** is a complex computer program used to control, assist or supervise all other programs that run on a computer system.

An **output device** is a piece of hardware for storing or displaying information, e.g. disk drive, monitor, printer.

**Output** is the information the computer gives out in response to input.

**Peripherals** are various attachments to the computer, e.g. keyboard, monitor, disk drive, printer, mouse.

**Personal data** consists of information about a living individual, including character references, but excluding any intentions of the data user in respect of that individual. The individual must be identifiable from the data. If the data does not contain a name, but contains a code number from which the data user can identify the individual, it is personal data.

**Pixel** is the pictorial element, a 'dot' on the screen. The fewer the pixels on screen, the larger they will be. Smaller pixels produce a higher resolution image on the screen.

**Pointer** is another name for cursor. The pointer changes its shape. Sometimes it looks like an arrow, sometimes like a vertical bar and at other times like a plus sign, hourglass, etc.

**Pointing** means placing the mouse pointer over a specific item or area on the screen.

**Ports** are connection points between computers and external devices such as printers.

**Program Group** is a collection of programs and documents represented by an icon.

A **program** is a series of detailed instructions written in a computer language that tells the computer what to do, e.g. a program might tell the computer to sort a list of names alphabetically.

**Program Manager** manages all activities when programs are being run under the Windows environment.

**PROM** is short for programmable read only memory. It is the same as ROM except that it is programmed by the user instead of the manufacturer.

**RAM.** Short for random access memory, a form of temporary internal storage whose contents can be retrieved and altered by the user; also called read-and-write memory.

**Read**, in computer language, means to load data from a storage medium, such as a disk, into the computer memory (RAM).

**Record.** In the context of a database each card is called a record.

**Registers** are locations in the computer's memory that can be accessed much more quickly than the general RAM.

**ROM** is short for read only memory. It is a permanent internal memory containing data or operating instructions that can be read but not altered by the user.

The **root directory** is the main directory on the disk. All other directories on the disk are branches from this main directory, or sub-branches.

A **shell** is a computer program that holds and manipulates the data constituting the knowledge base.

**Silicon** is an abundant semi-conducting element from which computer chips are made.

**Software**, broadly speaking, refers to the programs which provide the driving force of all computing systems. There are two types: (a) operating systems software and (b) applications software.

A **spell checker** is a computer program which allows the user to check that every word in a document is spelt correctly. Only the more expensive word processing packages have this facility.

A **spreadsheet** is an electronic sheet with horizontal rows and vertical columns forming cells at each point of intersection. Words, figures and formulae can all be added to the cells and calculations can be performed with the minimum of effort.

A **subdirectory** is a branch of a directory. This directory may itself be a branch of another directory. For example, in Figure 7.2, Reports is a subdirectory of Mydata. Mydata is a subdirectory of Winword. Winword is a subdirectory of D:\.

**TTNS (The Times Network Systems)** provides a multi-faceted communications and information service through the medium of information technology. It is a service to education as a whole.

**WAN** refers to a network of computers located far afield. It is an abbreviation for wide area network.

**Windows** can be described as a collection of programs, or suite of software, written for personal computers and published by Microsoft. It is sometimes referred to as a GUI (graphical user interface).

A **word processor** can be thought of as similar to a typewriter. To use it text must be typed in from the keyboard. However, it offers several advantages over the traditional typewriter.

**WORM** is an acronym for Write Once Read Many times. This is like the CD-ROM except that the user can enter his or her own data, but only once.

**Write**, in computer language, means to save data on to a storage medium, such as a disk.

**WYSIWYG** is an acronym for What You See Is What You Get. The way the document appears on the screen display closely resembles the way it will appear on paper when it is printed. An invaluable feature of a good word processing package.

# REFERENCES AND BIBLIOGRAPHY


Anderson, R. G. (1993) Data Processing Volume 1. Principles and Practice, 7th edn. London: Pitman.

Ball, M. J. and Hannah, K. J. (1984) Using Computers in Nursing. Virginia: Reston Publishing.

Barber, B. (1983) Computers need nursing. In M. Scholes, Y. Bryant and B. Barber (eds), The Impact of Computers on Nursing. Amsterdam: Elsevier Science Publishers, pp 24–33.

Bolwell, C. (1991) Directory of Educational Software for Nursing, 4th edn. New York: National League for Nursing, and Athens, OH: Fuld Institute for Technology in Nursing Education.

Bryant, J., Roberts, J. and Windsor, P. (eds) (1987) Current Perspectives in Health Computing. London: British Computer Society.

Chellen, S. (1994) A Study of attitudes of professional nurses and midwives towards computerisation in clinical settings and their expressed needs. MEd dissertation.

Chellen, S. and Jones, K. (1992) Chellen–Jones technique for the assessment of learning environments. A research project.

Cook, M. (1982) Using computers to enhance professional practice. Nursing Times, 78(37), 1542–5.

de Glanville, H. and Roberts, J. (eds) (1990) Current Perspectives in Health Computing. London: British Computer Society.

Eaton, N. (1991) Expert systems in nursing. Nursing Standard, 12(38), 32–3.

Greenhalgh and Co. Ltd (n.d.) Nurse Management Systems. A Guide to Existing and Potential Systems. Grasmere: Healthcare Management Consultants.

Greenhalgh, C. (1993) Its bark is worse than its byte. Nursing Standard, 7(15), 44–5.

Hamilton, M. (1993) Wireless data systems. What are they? What benefits are offered? Information Technology in Nursing and Other Health Care Professions, 5(4), 8–9.

Hannafin, M.J. and Peck, K. L. (1988) The Design, Development and Evaluation of Instructional Software. New York: Macmillan.

Henney, C. (1984) The use of computers for improvement and measurement of nursing care. In L. Willis and M Linwood (eds), Recent Advances in Nursing 10. Measuring the Quality of Care. Edinburgh: Churchill Livingstone, pp. 174–88.

HSE (1992) Working with VDUs. London: Health and Safety Executive.

Hudgings, C. and Meehan, N. (1984) SEINE: An Evaluation Tool for Computer Assisted Instruction. Computers in Nursing, 12, 35–7.

Koch, B. and Rankin, J. (1987) Computers and Their Applications in Nursing. London: Harper and Row.

Pawling, R. (1985) Computer applications in health professions. A report for Queen Margaret College, Edinburgh.

Procter, P. M. (1992) Nurses, Computers and Information Technology. London: Chapman and Hall.

Scarpa, R., Smeltzer, S. and Jasion, B. (1992) Attitudes of Nurses Toward Computerization: A Replication. Computers in Nursing, 10, 72–80.

Solomon, A., Solomon, S. and Bitton, P. (updated regularly) Dr Solomon's Anti-Virus Toolkit. Berkhamsted: S and S International Limited.

Starling, P. (1988) Current Perspectives in Health Computing. London: British Computer Society.

Stronge, H.J. and Bradt, A. (1985) Assessment of Nursesí Attitudes Towards Computerization. Computers in Nursing, 3 (4), 154–8.

Tanenbaum, A. S. (1984) Computer Networks, 2nd edn. Engelwood Cliffs, NJ: Prentice-Hall International.

Tanenbaum, A. S. (1984) Structured Computer Organization, 2nd edn. Engelwood Cliffs, NJ: Prentice-Hall International.

Van Bemmel, J. H. (1987) Computers assisted care in nursing – computers at the bedside. Computers in Nursing, 5(4), 232–5.

Vedera, S. (1989) Applied Expert Systems. Wilmslow: Sigma Press.

Walker, M. and Schwartz, C. (1984) What Every Nurse Should Know About Computers. Philadelphia: J. B. Lippincott.

# RECOMMENDED FURTHER READING


Ashworth, P. (1987) Technology and machines – bad masters but good servants. Intensive Care Nursing, 3(1), 1–2.

Burnard, P. (1991) Working with computers. Journal of District Nursing, 10(6), 18–19.

Chang, B. L. (1984) Adoption of innovations: nursing and computer use. Computers in Nursing, 2(6).

Greenhalgh, C. (1993). Shopping for systems. Nursing Standard, 7(18), 46–7.

Greenhalgh, C. (1993). Problems with nursing systems. Nursing Standard, 7(19), 46–7.

Hannah, K., Guillemin, F. and Conklin, D. N. (1986) Nursing Users of Computers and Information Science. Amsterdam: North Holland.

O'Desky, R. I. (1988) A neutral view of computing for nurses. In M. J. Ball et al. (eds), Nursing Informatics, Where Caring and Technology Meet. New York: Springer-Verlag, pp. 33–45.

Palmer, B. (1990) A smarter way of Nursing. Nursing Times, 86(9), 64–6.

Pawling, R. (1985) Computer applications in health professions, a report for Queen Margaret College, Edinburgh.

Peckitt, R. (1989) Computers in General Practice. Wilmslow: Sigma Press.

Rimmer, S. (1991) The Home Office Computer Book. New York: Sybex.

Sinclair, V. G. (1985). The Computer as a partner in health care instruction. Computers in Nursing, 3(5), 212–16.

# INDEX